Praise for Alexander Loyd

"Dr. Alex Loyd has the defining healing technology in the world today—it will revolutionize health. It is the easiest way to get well and stay well fast. Dr. Loyd may very well be the Albert Schweitzer of our time."
> —Mark Victor Hansen, coauthor of the
> Chicken Soup for the Soul books

"I have found no other process that is as elegantly simple, effortlessly learnable, inherently portable, profoundly effective, and fundamentally timeless. The highest commendation I can give is that I use it for myself, my family, and my patients."
> —Merrill Ken Galera, MD, medical director, the Galera
> Center, and former lead physician of Dr. Mercola's
> Natural Health Center

"You almost have to have a process like The Healing Code to change the wrong beliefs that are keeping you from the life and health you want."
> —Bruce Lipton, PhD, former cell biology
> researcher at Stanford University and author of the
> bestselling Biology of Belief

"This is a paradigm shift breakthrough, turns most conventional wisdom about how to achieve success on its head, and explains why so many things that have sounded good have failed to produce results over the last fifty years. I, for one, am 'all in'! I plan to live by and teach the Love Code from now on."
> —Janet Attwood, New York Times bestselling
> author of The Passion Test

"*The Memory Code* is packed with valuable information which offers a new perspective and a holistic approach to transforming your health by releasing and reengineering your stored memories. Dr. Alex Loyd, renowned author, healer, and energy-healing pioneer, reveals how memories from your past may be affecting your health, your life, your relationships, and your success. This easy-to-follow, step-by-step code will guide you through modifying your damaging negative memories, as well as those you have inherited from your ancestors, while giving you a deeper understanding of how your memories affect your emotional and physical health. Highly recommended!"

—Dr. Bradley Nelson, author of *The Emotion Code: How to Release Your Trapped Emotions for Abundant Health, Love, and Happiness*

THE
MEMORY
CODE

THE
MEMORY
CODE

THE 10-MINUTE SOLUTION
FOR HEALING YOUR LIFE THROUGH
MEMORY ENGINEERING

Alexander Loyd, PhD, ND

GRAND CENTRAL
PUBLISHING

New York   Boston

Grand Central Publishing
Hachette Book Group
1290 Avenue of the Americas, New York, NY 10104
grandcentralpublishing.com
twitter.com/grandcentralpub

First edition: October 2019

Grand Central Publishing is a division of Hachette Book Group, Inc. The Grand Central Publishing name and logo is a trademark of Hachette Book Group, Inc.

The publisher is not responsible for websites (or their content) that are not owned by the publisher.

The Hachette Speakers Bureau provides a wide range of authors for speaking events. To find out more, go to www.hachettespeakersbureau.com or call (866) 376-6591.

Library of Congress Cataloging-in-Publication Data has been applied for.

ISBNs: 978-1-5387-6442-8 (hardcover), 978-1-5387-6443-5 (ebook)

Printed in the United States of America

LSC-C

10   9   8   7   6   5   4   3   2   1

To Mom.
My first memory is you giving your life for mine.
I love you!

CONTENTS

PART ONE
The Great Memory Malfunction

PART TWO
THE MEMORY ENGINEERING TECHNIQUE

A WORD TO THE READER

In this book, I'm going to share with you a new approach to healing and personal growth called memory engineering. It goes straight to the source of the issues that have been holding you back in life, whether they're physical, emotional, or practical, and enables you to overcome them—especially when nothing else has seemed to work.

For thirty years, I've believed that our memories are the source of nearly everything we think, feel, and do, as well as of our body chemistry. So, for thirty years, I have been trying to find a way to fix, heal, and edit problematic memories. I have by no means been alone. After thirty years of searching, testing, failing, breakthroughs, testing again, and tweaking, I believe I've finally found it.

In *The Memory Code*, I'm offering what I believe to be a credible theory about how our memories work and why they are the true source of our life issues, as well as a simple process that allows you to reengineer your memories and heal your biggest problem at the source.

But before we dive into this theory and use it to solve your own biggest problem, I'd like to offer a kind of disclaimer. Memory research is a very new field of study. There is no machine that can show us our memories, and so any scientific evidence you may hear about how your memories work is partial at best. I'm going to be citing some scientific studies to support my theory throughout the book, but in no way do I want to imply that these studies "prove" my theory. They simply provide partial support for what I have seen and known to be true over the past thirty years of practice.

In fact, I don't believe double-blind studies in general are always the gold standard for truth, and here's why.

One of the geniuses I've had the privilege of studying under was Roger Callahan, PhD. He was a clinical psychologist who had a booming practice in Beverly Hills for years, but, like me, he was frustrated he wasn't helping a lot of his clients the way he wanted to. He became the founder of energy psychology worldwide, and I studied under him one-on-one for about a year and a half. Here's a quote of his that I absolutely love:

> "Double-blind studies are designed to prove whether something works when nobody can tell if it works."

In other words, if something obviously works for others and does no harm, you don't always need a double-blind study to confirm it works. This is, of course, not the case when discussing a pharmaceutical, which can have so many other negative side effects that it's not obvious the positive will outweigh the negative. Sometimes most of the commercial is spent telling you this drug may cause you to have suicidal thoughts, destroy your liver and kidneys, or cause cancer. If you have something like that, then yes, get a double-blind study!

Most pharmaceutical drugs are actually biological poisons being engaged to destroy one ailment even if it means doing damage to other areas. The body does not recognize the drug when it's ingested and identifies it as harmful, but then the drug essentially overpowers the body to create the intended effect, instead of working in harmony with the body's healing systems.

The current opioid epidemic in America, which many believe was fueled by the widespread prescribing of narcotics like OxyContin (oxycodone) without knowledge (or perhaps regard) for the negative effects, is just one obvious example. What seemed safe or proven wasn't really safe or proven, even in double-blind tests.

Several years ago I saw a doctor interviewed on *Larry King Live!* on the topic of vitamins. Twenty years ago, the doctor said, mainstream medicine was certain that the only benefit of vitamins was "expensive urine," while today doctors recommend vitamins to almost everybody. Why? "Because now we know it works," said the doctor.

Well, they always worked! And many people knew they worked before any studies "proved" they worked, took vitamins, probably received real benefits from them, and were mocked by the medical establishment until a double-blind study came out "proving" they worked.

Just because a double-blind test can't prove it doesn't mean it's not true. Did gravity not exist before Sir Isaac Newton discovered it? Did electricity not exist before Thomas Edison discovered the lightbulb? Did germs not exist before Louis Pasteur discovered them? Of course they did! They affected us just as much before science proved their existence.

Here's something else to consider. Professors have told me there's never in the history of the world been a double-blind study on counseling. Why? Because it's unethical. You'd have to give appropriate counseling to one group and inappropriate counseling to the other, which licensed counselors are not allowed to do.

How many people out there are saying, "There are no double-blind studies, so counseling has no validity in any situation"? I agree with the people who say that it very often does not deliver the results you wanted—that's why I shifted away from it. But I promise you, there are thousands of stories of people who have had their entire life turned around by good counseling and therapy.

My friend Jimmy Netterville, MD, a neurosurgeon at Vanderbilt Medical Center, said it best. Several years ago, we found ourselves sitting next to each other at a fund-raising dinner. He asked me about my work, and I told him that it had to do with energy medicine, and I explained a little bit about it. By this point I'd learned what sort of reaction to expect, and I said he probably thought that was crazy.

But he surprised me. He said, "No, no, no!" and he grabbed a dinner napkin and drew a line about six inches long. He said, "Alex, if this line is all knowledge that exists in the world about health, I believe we probably know about one inch of it. How arrogant and foolish it would be of me to say that what you're doing couldn't be in that other five inches—especially since there's such a history of medical science saying something is ridiculous and later being proven wrong."

Then he said something I'll never forget. "If it's helping people and not doing harm—I tell my patients to try it and come to me and tell me about it if it helps, so I can try it and see if it can help some of my other patients."

That pretty much sums up what I believe about memory engineering. It's helping people and not doing harm, so why not try it? In my opinion, there is no way it won't become a big deal in the future, because the issues it addresses are so critical to every single person on the planet. But right now, some of it is beyond that inch science has the tools to prove with double-blind studies.

And you must understand, I am not against the scientific method, double-blind studies, or standard medicine. If I get hit by a truck and am lying on the ground bleeding, don't do energy medicine on me; take me to the emergency room! But for many things in the natural and energy health field, there are no medical tests for what is being treated. The Memory Engineering Technique I'm going to teach you works on one thing: your memories, and mainly the unconscious ones.

It may very well take twenty years until we go from "this is pseudo-science" to "everybody needs to do this." As for you, you've got minutes a day to lose and twenty years to gain.

INTRODUCTION:
REMEMBERING THE REAL YOU

We don't see things as they are;
we see them as we are.
—Anaïs Nin

The date was July 7, 1959. The day of my birth—and of my mother's death.

My parents had been waiting for nine months, all the time knowing what was coming. They hadn't even meant to get pregnant again, and when they did, the doctors all told my mother one thing: "Abort. Save yourself."

So what sort of woman was my mother? A full-blooded German who raised her kids on polka music and spoiled them rotten with her cooking. A woman loved—in reciprocation—by everyone in town. A woman of such relentless and forceful empathy that she routinely outsold top businessmen in Chicago by going door-to-door peddling silverware, who furnished our home with prizes from her employer, and whose funeral, when it occurred, would be attended by dozens of former customers—now her friends.

The doctors informed this woman that her only option was to sacrifice my life for hers, and with tremendous fear, but without hesitation, she refused.

My birth should have been on the Fourth of July—

Independence Day. But my dad was in the fireworks business and had to work. They delayed the birth so that he could be there for it and, in all likelihood, say goodbye to his wife. I've always felt a little annoyed with him for that. I grew up in the family business. How perfect would it have been for a fireworks salesman to have a July 4 birthday? But looking back, I wonder what it must have meant to my mom. *Three more days to live.*

For nine months she carried me. I was a paradoxical child, the subject of both complete, unconditional love and complete, abject terror. In those final three days, she lay there in intense pain, waiting to give me her last and greatest gift.

But then: my mother didn't die. The doctors told her she would, she was prepared to do it for my sake, she had lived her life for most of a year thinking, *I'm going to die, I'm going to die, I'm going to die!* Yet when the time came, it didn't happen. So why did I call July 7, 1959, her death day?

Because even though the event didn't happen, it had become real to me. I was born under the specter of fear. Her image of that fictional event had replayed over and over in her mind for the entire nine months I was in her womb. *I'm going to die, I'm going to die, I'm going to die.* She passed that image and belief down to me so that I, too, believed I would die.

Even after my mother and I survived the birth, the danger wasn't over for me. I refused to swallow the food they gave me and lost several pounds within the first few days. The doctors put me in intensive care, but they couldn't make me eat, and I just kept getting worse. Beliefs like this affect all of us, but I think infants are especially vulnerable to them, because they don't yet have any conscious awareness to resist them. I believed I would die, and who could tell me otherwise?

I would have obeyed that programming I'd been born with, if not, once again, for my mother.

Against the advice of the doctors, she picked me up from the incubator and took me home. The doctors said, "He'll die if you leave the hospital." She responded, "He'll die if he stays." So we left.

For the next few days, she sat up with me twenty-four hours a day—holding me, singing to me, telling me she loved me, all the while trying to get me to eat. Although she may not have known it in so many words, she went to war with the fearful memory that was telling me I was going to die. She bombarded me with totally opposing experiences and images: *I love you, I love you, I love you.*

Eventually, love won, as love will. I began to swallow my food, and soon after that I was back to being healthy. But I continued to feel the repercussions of this story throughout my entire life—both good and bad. On one hand, I experience very strong affection, empathy, or love for someone that prompts me to help them, listen to them, or maybe just act as a friend. I believe this came from my birth experience, and it has become one of my greatest strengths.

On the other hand, I often experienced anxiety and had no idea where it was coming from, so I would usually assign it to whatever was happening that I didn't like. But it wasn't my circumstances causing my anxiety. It was my birth memories. How do I know? Only when I healed my memories related to my mother's health condition and my birth did my anxiety go away.

Powerful negative memories don't just go away once the event is over. Recent studies have proven that even when you're not consciously thinking about them, they can still affect you 24/7.

As a result, nearly everyone, for reasons they probably don't understand, believes and feels something their brains interpret as the danger of dying. They might not use that language—they might say, "This drives me crazy!" or "This is killing me!" or "I'm dying here!" Or they may simply feel a sense of panic or anxiety. But as far as the brain is concerned, it all amounts to the same thing: a constant undercurrent of stress that we can't release running through our daily lives.

Most of us are in a state of stress the majority of the time. Physiologically, the stress response means something is threatening our life, and therefore we go into fight, flight, or freeze mode to save our physical life. The problem is that we experience the stress response when we see a medical bill in the mailbox, or when the grocery store is out of our favorite snack, or if someone looks at us strangely. If you were stressed by a high medical bill, for example, and I asked you if you thought that hospital bill was literally going to kill you, your conscious mind would say, "That's crazy—of course not! I'm just a little stressed. No problem." But your unconscious mind—or what I will be calling our heart—is saying otherwise.

This is what I'm talking about when I say that everyone today is effectively living in an illusion: our bodies and mind live in a perpetual state of fear even when there is nothing in our environments to be afraid of. In this book, we're going to take a deeper dive into what the stress response was really intended for, how it began malfunctioning, and how that started a domino effect of malfunctioning in most areas of our lives—so that nearly everyone today is effectively living in an illusion. Yet even though this illusion has a huge, often negative impact on our lives, almost nobody seems to know it exists.

My birth story may sound extreme. Here's another example of how this illusion has a practical effect on our everyday life experience.

Mary, an attractive forty-three-year-old woman, sat down in my counseling office. Everything about her, down to the clothes, hair, and makeup, said success, the sort of person who would immediately make you think, *Yeah, she has it all together.*

However, Mary was distraught. Nothing was wrong, exactly. According to her own words, she was married to a good man, and although they weren't rich, they had everything they needed: a nice three-bedroom, two-bathroom house; good schools for their kids; extracurricular activities and friends they enjoyed. Yet the life Mary had envisioned as a girl had somehow turned into a life of "have tos."

She had tried various mood enhancers, both natural and prescription. Some helped and some didn't, but nothing really changed her basic outlook on life.

I asked about her childhood, and she told me she hadn't experienced anything abusive, although she did feel her mother had been hard on her most of the time, and her dad had been somewhat absent. Not so different from anyone else she knew.

When I asked if there was anything she looked forward to, her answer was going to bed or watching a few hours of mindless TV by herself.

Finally, I asked what she would most like to do, right now, if there were no repercussions. She answered me with tears in her eyes: "Drive to California and start over."

But Mary already knew she wasn't going to drive to California and start over. In fact, that was why she was in my counseling office: she loved her family, so she had resigned herself to a mediocre life, using most of her energy just to get through each day. She only wanted to see if I could help her cope better.

Not long afterward, a different woman came to my counseling office. She was also forty-three years old, had two kids, a husband doing well in his career, and a typical American middle-class lifestyle. She had had a somewhat overbearing mother and somewhat absent father.

But this woman was not in my office because she wanted to drive to California and start over. On the contrary, she *loved* her life!

This woman's life had far surpassed her childhood expectations, but not necessarily in the ways she would have guessed. It wasn't that she had more money, or more free time, or more anything, really, except maybe more love, gratitude, and contentment.

Throughout her day, she wasn't focused on just getting through it; she lived in and enjoyed each moment. Instead of going to bed or watching TV, her favorite time of day was waking up in the morning to be with her family.

In fact, I'd have to say she was one of the happiest, most content people I've ever had sit in my counseling office!

This woman wasn't there for counseling. She was there to say thank you. You see, it was Mary, six months later.

Nothing in her circumstances had changed. She still had the same family history, the same husband, the same kids, the same house—basically the same life. The only thing that had changed was how she *felt* about those circumstances. She felt good about herself and her life. She was happy; six months ago, she hadn't been.

As you think about your own life, which version of Mary's life do you most relate with?

You may be wondering, *If her circumstances didn't change, what could have possibly altered her feelings so dramatically?*

It wasn't her physiology, her brain chemistry, her thoughts, her emotions, or even her beliefs. It was something deeper, the same thing that shaped my life from the moment I was born.

It was her memories.

TREATING THE SYMPTOMS, NOT THE SOURCE

Okay, let's start with a little survey.

Would you like to change your life in any of the following ways:

- Have more energy
- Make more money

- Experience less anxiety and more peace
- Feel more joyful
- Feel more passionate and excited about life
- Have better work-life balance
- Break an addiction
- Feel less trapped and experience more freedom
- Be more successful at work, or change careers
- Get better sleep
- Have more "me" time
- Have more confidence or a higher sense of self-worth
- Lose weight
- Exercise more
- Improve your diet
- Heal a health issue
- Have a closer relationship with your spouse or significant other
- Spend more time with your friends or make new ones
- Get along better with your family
- Find clarity about your life purpose
- Leave a legacy of significance
- Help a loved one with a significant need

I have worked with hundreds of people over the years who had a problem but didn't have the first clue where it was coming from. They would eventually blame it on something in their current circumstances, which was almost never the true cause, and doing so eventually led to a vicious cycle or addiction.

For instance, Pete had an anger problem. He would typically get angry three or four times a day, out of nowhere. It was about to break up his marriage, and he was at his wits' end. He had received a little counseling, tried some drugs for anxiety, and in his words "tried really hard" to control it—but he couldn't. He would get mad at work, at home, on the way home in traffic—you name it. Whenever something didn't go his way, he got irritated or angry. He believed the problem was in his circumstances, and the solution was to somehow control his reaction to his circumstances.

But as we worked through the process you'll learn in this book, Pete discovered that the real source of his anger was not being able to live up to his dad's expectations and feeling rejected by him. Pete had even become a medical doctor to try to impress his dad, but nothing ever seemed to work. After about six weeks, he healed his memory of his dad's rejection, his anger problem immediately became a non-issue, and he was also able to heal his relationship with his wife. The cycle was broken.

If you're struggling to make permanent, positive change in *any* area of your life, it might be because you're treating the symptoms, not the source. This book is going to help you diagnose the *real* source of your problem—and likely fix it for good.

Now let me ask you a quick question, one I might ask if you came to my office.

Let's say you're at home, and water starts flooding your kitchen floor. You don't live anywhere close to water, and it's not raining outside. What would you do first: start cleaning up the water on the floor or would you turn off the water to the house?

This is a much more important question than you might think. Most people, perhaps after a minute, would go turn off the water to the house and then start wiping up the floor. Wiping up the floor without stopping the water would be crazy, right?

Over the past eighty years or so, the psychological, self-help, spiritual, and medical worlds have offered a variety of theories on fixing the source of our problems. At certain times, some have been more popular than others, but you can still find books and experts claiming any one of these as the true source even today:

• *Circumstances.* Think of SMART goals (Specific, Measurable, Achievable, Relevant, and Time-based), vision boards, and the advice to "just do it." Change your circumstances, change your life.

• *Behavior.* Act "as if." Do the right thing, and the feelings will follow. Change your behavior, change your life.

• *Physiology and brain chemistry.* If you can find the right drug or supplement, follow the optimal diet, or meditate long or often enough, you'll start feeling good about yourself. Change your chemistry, change your life.

• *Conscious thoughts.* Understand the truth and think the right way about it. If you just realize how fortunate you are compared to your neighbor, you'll start feeling better. Substitute positive thoughts for negative ones. Change your thoughts, change your life.

- *Conscious beliefs.* Your beliefs are an even stronger, deeper combination of thoughts and feelings that define what is most important about you. Change your beliefs, change your life.

- *Emotions.* Emotional mastery is a hot topic today with a variety of techniques. Change your emotions, change your life.

All of these solutions provide wonderful insight about the way we work as humans and often do make us feel better...for a while. The problem is that after eighty years of personal development solutions, people are hungrier for solutions than ever. How can that be?

Because all of these solutions are just different ways of wiping the water off the floor. If you work hard enough and constantly enough, you might actually get ahead of the leak. Every once in a while, you might look around, enjoy your dry floor, and think the solution worked.

But you still haven't fixed the leak in your kitchen. That's why you're so tired all the time! You're using all your energy to clean up without stopping the flood at its source! Of course, any of these solutions can still be better than nothing, but even if you could follow them all at once, and follow them perfectly, *you still wouldn't stop the water from coming in.*

That's exactly what this book will show you how to do. Only recently have we discovered a deeper cause for our feelings, beyond our circumstances, behavior, brain chemistry, thoughts, emotions, and even beliefs.

Our memories.

MEMORIES MAKE US WHO WE ARE

You may be skeptical. I understand. Let me explain what I mean.

First of all, I'm not talking about your ability to remember, to consciously recall facts you've learned or events that happened to you. I'm also not referring to "process memories," such as learning to ride a bike, walk, or play Ping-Pong. When people say, "It's like riding a bike," they're referring to something you'll never forget. Process memories rarely degrade or develop errors over time.

I'm talking about what I call your *source memories*, created from your life experience, your imagination, and even the subconscious experiences and impressions inherited from many generations of ancestors and passed down to you.

Source memories are a different animal. They are the lens through which you see yourself and everything in the world. Everything that happens to you runs through the source memories of your life and ancestry to determine your thoughts, feelings, beliefs, actions, and even the hormones and physiology of your body. Unfortunately, they're also prone to errors, as you'll discover in part 1.

However, process and source memories have one thing in common: each new related memory builds on the previous one. When a baby learns to walk, does she just stand up and start walking? No, she tries and falls about five thousand times first! Each of those falls creates a memory that eventually leads to the ability to walk—the feel of balancing, of using her leg muscles, etc. Every new memory builds on the previous one until the baby finally has all the memories needed to successfully stand up and then to walk. Walking requires the whole sequence of standing-and-walking–related memories, which may be in the hundreds or even thousands. If any memories in the chain were deleted, skipped, or altered incorrectly, the baby may never learn.

Neuroscientist and professor Antonio Damasio has shown that at the root of every thought, belief, feeling, and action is an *image*. These images are what I'm talking about when I use the term "source memories" and, from now on, simply memories. These images, or memories, come from:

- **Events in our own lives**, including both those we consciously remember (like our high school prom, our first day at our job, or what we ate for lunch yesterday) and those we don't consciously remember (like being born, or how our parents spoke to us when we were infants and toddlers).
- **Our imagination**, such as when we daydream about our upcoming vacation or worry that our loved one will get into a car accident.
- **Previous generations**, such as trauma experienced by a parent or grandparent, or by their parents or grandparents—like what I was exposed to in the womb.

The truth is that our memories make us who we are in virtually every way—and new studies are revealing this more and more every day. We come into this world with a set of inherited memories, and from the time we're born, we're interpreting everything through the lens of those memories and making new ones that build on top of one another, so that we learn and develop strategies to stay safe.

When we make our memories, we're making our life—or, in some cases, our death.

THE MEMORY MALFUNCTION

Here's the problem. Memories that trigger our "this is going to kill me" interpretation and response (otherwise known as the stress response or fear response) are prioritized above all other memories or beliefs, whether these memories are from our personal experience, from our imagination, or inherited. When anything even remotely related to this memory occurs, we have a "this is going to kill me" response, whether it's related to our physical safety, or our identity, security, and relationships.

Why is that a problem? Don't we want our memories to keep us safe? Well, it's not a problem—if our memories always tell us the truth about what could truly kill us. But what if they don't?

We tend to think our memories are like audio and visual recordings of what actually happens to us, but they're not. As we'll also discuss in part 1, our real-life experiences are filtered through the lens of our danger memories first—and we've seen what can happen when those memories are wrong. For so many of my clients, one single negative memory "screwed them for life"; their words, not mine—although I know how they feel.

For example, one guy I worked with felt like he could never live up to his dad. When he was fourteen, he was running for class president, and because his dad had experience successfully running for office, he was asking his son some questions to help him prepare. At some point, after one of his answers, his dad chuckled and said, "You must think you're me. Let me tell you something: you're not me, and that's not going to work."

Those words changed the course of his life. For twenty years, he was haunted by the sense that he would never be as good as his father. He saw everything even remotely related to that situation through the lens of that memory, which would create a new negative memory, which created a new one, and so on. And of course, all those related memories were sending off unconscious stress signals 24/7.

Later, when my client asked his father about it, he discovered that his father meant his son was *better* than he was. That memory had crucial errors in it—the comment was meant as a compliment, but he received it as criticism, telling him, "I'm not good enough to do anything." It was a memory that shaped almost everything in his life, and it was all based on a misunderstanding.

Other times, there is no misunderstanding. Growing up, my dad and I had a very close, loving relationship. But when I was about twelve years old, he was diagnosed with heart disease, which was almost like a death sentence back then. Out of the blue, one day my dad started hitting me over and over again, yelling, "You're never going to amount to anything!"

That event actually happened—my dad really did beat me that day, and he really did say I would never amount to anything. My memory of that event—and all the subsequent memories seen through that lens—would negatively shape me for the next fifteen years.

My daily mood and even my personality shifted after that day. I talked less, felt worse about myself as a person, did worse in school, and started getting into trouble in ways I never had before. The biggest change was my anger. Before, I had never really had any anger issues, but all of a sudden I had a hair-trigger temper. I had always sung out loud around home a lot, and I completely quit singing. It was like the joy was sucked out of my heart and replaced with anger.

I didn't consciously connect the incident with my dad to the changes in how I felt about myself. I didn't know why I felt these things or felt compelled to act in different, dark ways. I realize now that I had largely suppressed that memory because of its pain, so I didn't know why I was helpless to do and feel what I wanted to do and feel. I was confused, in pain, and helpless to treat the root of what had started me down this path. This pattern basically continued until my wife kicked me out of the house at age twenty-seven, which led to the biggest spiritual transformation of my life (more about that later).

How about Mary, the client I mentioned earlier? For her, the issue wasn't her current circumstances (her marriage, her children, her house, even her current relationship with her mother), but her memories of her overbearing mother created during her childhood.

One of these memories was of doing the dishes and her mom berating her for not doing them the way she had instructed. What Mary kept thinking was that she had done them exactly like she had done them the day before, and her mom had said, "Great job, honey." This was a frequent experience, whether it was how she kept her room, or the way she did her makeup, or the boys she dated. One day something would be okay, and the next day it wouldn't be. Her mom's responses were inconsistent and personally demeaning, and Mary couldn't find solid ground.

She didn't realize it, but those defining memories shaped how she felt about herself and her life to the present day. She often felt she had to constantly pretend to be someone she wasn't, and that what other people thought about her was critical and she needed to be guarded at all costs. At the end of a berating, her mom would always say, "Now, you know I just want what's best for you, honey, and I just want you to have a better life than me." But it didn't feel that way to Mary.

Those memories caused her to view every experience through a lens that distorted everything. They were why she found herself in survival mode, trying to numb herself to her constant stress through sleep or mindless TV, and fantasizing about driving to California and never coming back—despite the fact that, from the outside, her life looked secure and even ideal to most that knew her.

In all four of these situations, the problems began when we connected an *event* with our *identity*—that because x happened, we're bad and not good. Or that because y happened, we'll never be loved. Or that because z happened, we will never be successful.

Conclusions like these are never true. Even the worst abuse in your past has nothing to do with your ability to be safe, secure, or have relationships now (assuming you are not currently in a life-or-death or abusive situation), or your value *ever*. But these memories create illusions for us that limit or even prevent us from being able to move past them.

When we accept these wrong conclusions as truth and continue through life thinking, feeling, and acting according to them, *we are living a lie!* And we will be for as long as we accept as true that which is not true.

This is the extraordinary power of the mind. In the German language, the word *imagination* has two meanings. One is to daydream, while the other is to create.

We have all daydreamed. As a child, I used to imagine winning Wimbledon and the US Open every year. While those particular daydreams never came true, later in my life I discovered that my imagination had the power to release me from the shackles of my pain and fear. We all have the tools that we need to change our lives forever, to create our absolute best life using the tool of our image maker. Using it to create memories of success, health, great relationships, and love can transform your internal life beyond your imagination.

REMEMBERING THE REAL WORLD

I hope by this time you're wondering if errors in your memories—from your own life, from your imagination, or from past generations—are holding you back. If so, here are two simple diagnostics.

1. Do you generally wake up each morning feeling like you just need to get through the day? Do you spend most days battling stress, anxiety, and "have tos," and feeling like something's missing in your life?
2. Do you get angry sometimes (or experience any emotion or feeling in the anger family, such as irritation, frustration, etc.)? When you look back, are you ever embarrassed about or unsure why you had the reaction that you did?

If either of these fit you, you're not alone. The vast majority of people today fall into these categories. Unless you're currently in profound physical or emotional danger right now, these everyday struggles are a sign that you have memories negatively influencing your life and wrongly making you feel bad. You don't have to keep feeling this way, and maybe you never should have in the first place.

The rest of this book will explain how our memory has evolved, or in this case devolved, and how you can travel back in time to change your past—if not in minutes, then typically in a matter of days or a few weeks.

My first book, *The Healing Code*, showed you how to heal the source of your health problems, and *The Love Code* showed you how to heal the source of your success blockages. *The Memory Code* will show you how to heal the source of any problem, based on cutting-edge research and a brand-new six-step, ten-minute process. You'll learn how to turn off the water rather than become an expert in cleaning it up, so you can use all that extra energy to live and feel the best life you can—for yourself, your loved ones, and for the world.

But first, you have to make a choice.

In my experience (which is now supported by research we'll examine later in the book), well over 90 percent of all people carry a belief that is negatively affecting their life experience. More specifically, they have come to the wrong conclusions about critical aspects of their life and circumstances that have created these devastating beliefs.

I believe memory engineering is part of a new frontier of medicine and psychology. So if you want to live your best life, with full access to your energy and potential and talent, it's time to make your choice: Are you going to keep doing what you've always done and just endure the rest of your life? Or will you take the plunge for something better?

I work with people who want to go for it, or else I don't work with them! I assist people who, when they reach that moment of crisis, don't resign themselves to a life of survival. They want to reach that higher vista so badly that they're willing to leave behind everything they thought they knew. Because they want the whole truth and their very best life, not just what's easy. They want to go for it.

Do you want to go for it? If so, meet me in the next chapter, and we'll start this journey together.

PART ONE

The Great Memory Malfunction

CHAPTER ONE

How Humans Were Designed to Function (But Don't Anymore)

Because your memories drive your every thought, feeling, belief, action, and chemical reaction in your body, I want to make this very real for you.

Take a moment to remember your most recent really good day. When was it? What happened? Close your eyes and try to really experience it again—taste it, smell it, touch it, feel it—just for a minute or two.

Now, think about your last bad day. When was it? What happened? Taste it, smell it, touch it, feel it—go back there for a moment.

What made those days good or bad? What did you feel and think about each day's experiences?

If you're like most people, what made it a good or bad day was how you felt about the *external circumstances* at the time. Something great happened in your world, or something bad you were worried over turned out fine, and so you remember it—you "feel" it—as a great day. On the other hand, when something bad happened in your life, or something you really wanted to happen didn't, you remember that—you "feel" it—as a bad day.

While this is natural, the belief that your quality of life depends on your external circumstances is wrong. To put it bluntly, you're living a lie. And that lie is the root and source of the great majority of human suffering in this world.

What if I were to tell you that almost every day of your life could be a good day, regardless of what happened? Not that you could be the exception to the rule, but that *all humans were designed to experience a good day most every day?*

And that even when the infrequent real catastrophe occurs, you're designed to bounce back quickly and resume your previously consistent good days?

The fact that most people don't experience life this way is the result of a malfunction that has evolved in the brain over thousands of years—that malfunction I mentioned in the introduction and that I'll explain in the next few chapters. But when it seems like everyone around you has bad days or "blah" days more often than not, it's hard to believe that having a bad day is a malfunction—how could everybody be broken? But the truth is, almost everybody is. We think whether we have a good, bad, or so-so day is determined by our circumstances, and therefore there's no other choice, but that's just not correct. It's a glitch, an internal virus causing us to malfunction and experience the world through a broken filter. So, in this chapter, I want to begin by very briefly showing you how I believe human beings were designed to work.

WE ARE WIRED FOR LOVE—UNLESS WE'RE IN DANGER

According to cognitive neuroscientist Caroline Leaf, PhD, we have no mechanisms inside us—body, mind, or spirit—whose function is to create a negative experience or physiology.[1] The purpose of every human mechanism or process is to create a positive result. "For example, we have an area in the brain called the *corpus striatum* that seems to be involved in positive reinforcement. This wired-for-love system is designed to respond to calmness, peacefulness, and feeling good, [when we are] filled with self-confidence and esteem. When we do not feel safe, it does not get activated."[2]

Similarly, Rebecca Turner, PhD, of the University of California, San Francisco, and Margaret Altemus, MD, of Cornell University reported research that showed the feel-good hormone oxytocin is released when a person experiences love-based memories and relationships, as long as there are not too many fear-based memories.[3]

If we don't feel safe, a mechanism in the brain based in the hypothalamus releases a flood of chemicals to get us out of danger fast, so we can return to that "wired for love" state. We'll talk more about this mechanism later in the chapter.

In addition to this chemical positive default setting, there are two other features of the human experience that contribute to our overall positive default setting: the way our heart works and the way we're wired for relationships.

OUR LIFE EXPERIENCE IS GOVERNED BY THE HEART

More than three thousand years ago, King Solomon wrote in his Proverbs, "Guard your heart above everything else, for from it flow the issues of life." Here Solomon is not referring to our cardiological heart, but our spiritual heart—or what I will be simply referring to as "heart" from now on.

One of the friends I grew up with, Jimmy Netterville, is now a renowned neurosurgeon at Vanderbilt Medical Center. Here's what he told me about being a brain surgeon: "People are impressed, but really what I do is like cutting a bad piece of apple out—and most of the time it comes back! For some time I've thought that there has to be a better way."

I believe that same thing to be true about how we treat and try to heal from our emotional malfunctions. You can't solve the problem without addressing the source. And I believe the source of all our issues, like Solomon said, is found in the heart.

For the purposes of this book, I'd like to define some basic terms.
- Our conscious mind includes memories we can recall on demand.
- Our subconscious mind includes memories we may not remember on demand but that can impact and sometimes surface within our conscious mind.

- Our unconscious mind includes memories we don't know we have and may not even be able to consciously access.
- Our spirit is our essence, the eternal part of who we are.
- Our heart includes the unconscious, subconscious, conscience, spirit, and right brain.

The Delta-Theta Brainwave State

Studies show that it takes ten positive experiences to off-set one negative experience in childhood—yet studies also show that children experience ten negatives to one positive. That's certainly going to cause malfunctions, as we'll see later, but even here we come equipped with a mechanism that protects us from the effects of stress as children.

According to electroencephalogram (EEG) readings of adult brainwaves, adults can experience five different brainwave states: delta, theta, alpha, beta, and gamma. According to EEG readings of children's dominant brainwave states, during our first six years of life, we are primarily in a *delta* and/or *theta* brainwave state.[4]

In order of frequency, delta is the slowest brain-wave state, and in adults it occurs during deep, dream-less sleep.[5] However, children up to the age of two are able to experience delta while awake, and the result is their experiences instantly become part of their deepest programming.

Theta is the next brainwave state in terms of frequency, and it's characteristic of daydreaming or REM sleep (active dreaming).[6] Beginning at around age two, children shift primarily into the theta brainwave state while awake, which adults experience during light sleep or deep meditation. In children, it's characterized by creative thought and often combining the imaginary and physical worlds.[7]

Between the ages of six and twelve, children shift primarily into alpha, a relaxed state of learning and the transition into conscious, logical thought. In adults, it's experienced as mental rest and reflection.[8]

By about age twelve, our cerebral cortex has developed enough so that we can experience the beta brainwave state, characterized by self-awareness, logical thought, and conscious decision-making. If beta waves are high enough, this is also where we experience stress.[9]

In terms of development, that means we essentially have two brainwave stages: before beta and after beta. Up to the age of six or so, because our cerebral cortex hasn't developed to the point where we can experience conscious thinking and self-awareness, we have absolutely no filter: everything is instantly downloaded to our heart.

At the same time, as we're learning what it takes to survive as babies and children, our life-or-death response is going off all the time—for good reason. We are far more likely to die an accidental death during early childhood, so this system is built into us to ensure our literal physical survival.

As a child, I vividly remember not being able to sleep

because there was a monster in my closet looking at me, just waiting until I went to sleep so he could come out and get me. My parents had already checked the closet, as had my brother, but the monster was too sneaky for them. Now I was stuck. No one believed me, but if I went to sleep, I would be killed horribly.

A mother of a five-year-old told me this story: Her son had been wanting to learn to ride his bike without his training wheels, but whenever she took them off, he would give up after a couple of minutes. She finally asked him, "What do you think will happen if you fall off the bike?" He immediately answered (while wearing his helmet), "I'll die."

Even though there was no monster in my closet, and even though the little boy wasn't going to die if he fell off his bike, these beliefs weren't really malfunctions. At that age, our minds are supposed to overreact to any potential danger. The alternative is to underreact, which could mean we don't survive. That's why kids see almost everything as exaggerated. We don't have the knowledge database yet about what is safe or unsafe, so our feelings are magnified to compensate and keep us from danger.

But here's the beautiful part: because we can't shift into beta, *we can't experience the negative effects of chronic stress.* The delta-theta brainwave state is one of the best protective systems we have to keep our default experience positive, even at the age when we're legitimately driven by fear as we figure out which behaviors are safe and which aren't.

Luckily, we shift out of this stage eventually. Let's say you're at a party, and you see one of your friends drinking a soda. "Hey, could you pass me a soda, too?" you ask. "I'm sorry, this is the last one," they reply.

Would you throw yourself down on the floor and throw a tantrum? No! But that's exactly what a three-year-old might do. What would be a massive malfunction for you is a natural part of our survival mechanism as children.

Here's why this is important to us today: the strength of our fear memories is determined by the amount of adrenaline released during the event. Even if we think we haven't experienced any big traumas, everyone has a bucket of these delta-theta memories that act like traumas, because of the amount of adrenaline released. These memories also need to be healed with memory engineering.

Because they don't have the ability to rationalize yet, kids are great at calling this spade a spade: "I think I'll die!" As adults, if we feel afraid and don't know why, it very well may be a result of one of these delta-theta memories. But we rationalize and correlate our fear with some other external circumstance. This is a tragedy, because if we could just be honest, we could address and heal the source: *Yes, I "feel" like this traffic is going to kill me, so let me find and fix the memories at the source of this malfunction.*

Memories Are the Language of Our Heart

Images, not words, are the universal language. We see and interpret a picture at the speed of light; understanding the meaning of words is a slow, archaic process in comparison. Images are also the native language of our heart, our most basic form of communication on a cellular level.

This is also why I believe the heart includes our right brain: the right brain is where images and meaning reside. The functions of the right and left brain are well established. In 1982, Roger Sperry, PhD, won the Nobel Prize for his split-brain research. Patients were having epileptic storm seizures to the point where they couldn't function—they couldn't sleep, they couldn't eat, and some were dying. Dr. Sperry took dramatic action and severed the corpus callosum, which connects the left and right brain. His logic was that if he cut the connection, the storm seizures would stop.

He was right. The seizures did stop when he severed the corpus callosum. Severing the connection also caused some specific new problems, but overall, the patients were able to live relatively normal lives—certainly much better than before.

Then Dr. Sperry realized that he had a group of people unlike any that had existed before, and he decided to try a series of experiments. In one of his most famous experiments, he asked a patient who was hungry to sit down at a table with a bowl of food and a spoon. He asked the patient to cover his left eye, which meant the patient had no access to right-brain information about the objects on the table. Any response or behavior would come 100 percent from his left brain.

Dr. Sperry asked the person what he saw on the table. The person would say the word *spoon*, but after a few more questions, it was clear that he didn't know what a spoon was, what it was used for, or how to use it. Then Dr. Sperry told the patient to cover up his right eye, so that he was only accessing the right brain. The patient didn't know the word for "utensil" or say anything at all—he just picked up the spoon and started to eat.

In further experiments, when Dr. Sperry's split-brain patients were asked to operate without access to their right brain, he found that they couldn't trust, use wise judgment, cooperate (e.g., be part of a meaningful relationship), act or behave appropriately, exercise wisdom and healthy judgment, feel, or even think! Even when they were hungry, they couldn't pick up the spoon and eat.

Now that the functions of the left and right brain could be distinguished and isolated, the differences were clear: left-brain knowledge is communicated in words, and is logical, analytical, conceptual, and time-based. Right-brain knowledge is communicated in images, and is intuitive, holistic, feeling-based, and timeless.

Why am I going into such detail about the left and right brain? Because we live in a left-brain world. The left brain's purpose is kind of like the bumpers at the bowling alley. When we have an emotional overreaction to our circumstances because of the image the heart pulled up, the left-brain/conscious mind is supposed to say, "Stop everything, that's not right! There's something in my heart that needs attention, if I had a reaction like that."

While the right brain is all over the place, the left brain always has feet on the ground. You can't just let your heart do whatever it wants, because it almost always contains bad programming. At the same time, even if the left brain/ conscious mind was right all the time (which it's not), it is far too weak to control the images of the heart. Left and right are designed to work together in harmony, like two oars on a rowboat. If the oars aren't in harmony, you'll never reach the right destination.

Antonio Damasio, MD, PhD, one of the top experts in neuroscience today and professor and chair of the neuroscience department at the University of Southern California, has said, "Brains can have many intervening steps in the circuits mediating between stimulus and response, and still have no mind, if they do not meet an essential condition: the ability to display images internally and to order those images in a process called thought. (The images are not solely visual; there are also 'sound images,' 'olfactory images,' and so on.)" Imageless thought is impossible.

It's also important to note that memories and images do not reside in your brain alone: they are also written on the cells themselves. In *The Love Code*, I cited a study from Southwestern University that made national news, where the researchers said they had found the source of illness and disease. They called it *cellular memory*. According to their research, cells record their own experiences without the involvement of the brain, and these cellular memories may be the determining factor in whether we experience cancer, psychological trauma, addiction, depression, and other conditions. They also seem to affect the memories that do require our brain.[10]

Related to this idea of cellular memory is the field of

epigenetics, which studies the biological mechanisms that turns genes on or off. In his bestselling book *The Biology of Belief*, cell biologist and epigenetics pioneer Bruce Lipton, PhD, said, "The cell is like a camera. Whatever is in the environment, the membrane is like a lens, it picks up the image and sends that image to the nucleus where the database is. That's where the stored images are."[11]

I believe that what Lipton refers to as "stored images" the Southwestern researchers call "cellular memory," and Damasio refers to as "images" are all different slices of the same pie: what I'm calling source memories—the source of our life issues. We'll talk more about how these source memories work in the next chapter.

Whether you like it or not, the heart will take over at critical times in your life, as you'll see in the next section. We need to consciously cooperate with how we're made instead of trying to work against it all the time. When we try to work against how we're made, we're putting ourselves in constant stress. The only wise solution is to learn about it, work with it, and sit in the control seat, as this book will show you how to do.

The Life-or-Death Response

Science shows us that we're wired for love—until we enter a state of fear. Our heart is a finely tuned instrument that is programmed for survival, and it's equipped with certain safety features to get us out of danger fast. The first is the life-or-death response, commonly known as the stress response.

A few years ago, I was going through the airport, and in

my bag I had a light therapy device I was testing. It looked kind of like a little kid's toy wooden gun. No one would ever mistake it for a real gun after taking a quick look at it, but I was a little nervous about taking it through security.

I went through security, and nobody said a thing. I was relieved; I had a flight to catch! As I was putting my belt back on, I commented without really thinking, "You didn't find the thing that looks like a gun."

There were six guys surrounding me in two seconds. They grabbed me, took me to a room, and locked me in. Needless to say, I was scared.

After about twenty endless minutes, a man walked in.

"Okay, Dr. Loyd, explain to me what happened from your perspective," he asked in a kind and reasonable manner.

I told him about the device that I was carrying with me, which I hadn't checked in my luggage because I didn't want it to get lost. They did a background check on me and a thorough search of all my belongings. At the end of it, the officer concluded it was just a misunderstanding. Then he said, "Dr. Loyd, let me give you a piece of advice. Do not, under any circumstances, say the word 'gun' in an airport. Those guys who grabbed you— if they hear the word 'gun,' they have to grab you. They have no choice; they get in trouble if they don't."

That's a lot like the way our heart works. Its primary safety feature is the fear response, or what I like to call the "life-or-death" response, because that's exactly what it is. It's designed to get us out of life-threatening danger fast, even if it means overreacting—just like the men at the airport were trained to rush in the moment they heard the word "gun." The alternative, not rushing in and running the risk that someone could possibly get killed, just isn't worth it.

If something in your current circumstances resembles even loosely what your heart has defined as potentially life threatening, a match gets made, and your heart pulls your internal fire alarm. Your hypothalamus gets activated, your survival mechanism takes over your thoughts, feelings, and actions, and it gears your body up to run, fight, or hide with a flood of cortisol and adrenaline. In essence, the heart sends in the Fear Response Team and commands our conscious mind to go sit in the corner, saying, "We've got this one."

If your current circumstances *don't* seem relevant to anything that your unconscious has defined as life threatening, your conscious mind and conscience have reasonable control of your thoughts, feelings, and actions, based on whatever you decide in the moment. Because we are wired for love, our thoughts, feelings, and actions should naturally tend to be positive. (However, as you'll see in the next chapter, because of the devolution we've experienced in our memories, this is now no longer the case.)

When the life-or-death response turns on, the body is flooded with a stress hormone called cortisol. Excessive exposure has the following well-documented clinical results:

- Dumbs us down
- Makes us sick

- Drains energy
- Suppresses the immune system
- Increases pain
- Raises blood pressure
- Closes cells
- Causes fear, anger, depression, confusion, shame, and worth and identity issues

As we'll see later, long-term exposure to cortisol can eventually result in a state akin to shock, where we feel unable to deeply experience anything. It's the "freeze" part of fight/flight/freeze.

When we're in a love-based state, love-based memories cause the release of oxytocin and other chemicals into the brain, which have these results:

- Enhances relationships
- Increases parental bonding
- Results in love, joy, and peace
- Increases immune function
- Reduces stress
- Lowers blood pressure
- Opens cells
- Stimulates human growth hormone
- Modulates appetite, healthy digestion, and metabolism
- Stimulates relaxation
- Stimulates higher neurological activity[12]

Let me give you an example of how significant the stress response is: according to the research of Bruce Lipton, stress is the only way you can get sick or contract a disease. Lipton conducted research at Stanford University to determine what causes healthy cells to become diseased and vice versa. In one of his experiments, when he removed cancer cells from an individual and put them in a petri dish, the cells became healthy all by themselves. After continued research, he concluded that the physical environment of the cell (i.e., the patient) caused the disease. After even further research, Lipton concluded that the key determinant in the environment was stress. The fear response functioned like a chemical "disease switch" for the cell: if the fear response was on, the cell "closed," and disease began. If the fear response was not turned on, the cell was open and, according to Lipton, the cell did not get sick.

In fact, Lipton says that 95 percent of all disease and illness is caused by stress. If 95 percent of all disease and illness is caused by the environment of the cell, what about the other 5 percent? Lipton found that the other 5 percent was due to nature—a genetic mutation passed down from your ancestors. But can you guess the cause of that genetic mutation? Stress. According to Lipton, stress was the cause of unmasking that genetic disease gene in the first place. His conclusion is that virtually 100 percent of illness and disease comes from stress, which he says comes from wrong internal beliefs, and I would say those wrong internal beliefs come from errors in your memories.

So is disease and illness a result of nature or nurture? The answer is *both*. But the "nurture," or the environment, we're talking about isn't nutrition or clean air or any other external characteristic. The key issue is *internal stress*. If you're stressed, your cells will get sick, because the first thing stress does is turn off your immune system.

That's another reason I will insist on calling the fear or stress response our "life-or-death" response. It's not only a sign that you have a memory telling you your circumstances are going to physically kill you; the stress response itself will literally kill you—slowly, gradually, but inevitably.

You have an immune system for a reason: it's supposed to work on your behalf! If you don't turn your immune system back on, you could eat the cleanest diet and live in the purest environment on earth, and you still wouldn't be able to avoid every single threat.

If you're *not* stressed, your immune system is fully operational, and your cells are capable of resisting and healing any disease or illness—even cancer, according to Lipton's studies.

That seems to lead to an amazing conclusion: healing from stress is the best preventive medicine available. It's completely free and always accessible to every single one of us. This research has been around for decades. Why isn't this being taught in every public school and university around the world?

So, if stress turns off our immune system, what turns off stress? Lipton believed the source of stress was our beliefs, but as you know, I believe the source of stress is one step deeper than beliefs: our source memories. Every belief is an interpretation of our cumulative memories about that issue, with the negative memories receiving much more weight. So even if we have 99 positive or neutral memories about a particular issue, we could still easily have a negative "belief" about that issue if a lot of adrenaline was released during one experience. This may make it seem like we are slaves to our memories, but do not fear: we can heal and resolve them, which you'll learn to do in part 2.

Psychological Adaptation

The good news is that even if we experience long-term stress, we are built with a wonderful safety feature called *psychological adaptation*. This mechanism helps you adjust positively to virtually any circumstance. Years ago, I saw a documentary that mentioned a study on two groups of people: the first group had just won the lottery and become millionaires overnight, and the second group had just been in a catastrophic accident and became paraplegics for life.

Both groups were given all kinds of physical and emotional tests, and at the start of the study, the lottery-winner group scored much happier on every single measure, both physical and non-physical, compared to the other group. There was about as big a difference as you could imagine. Six months later, the tests were administered again. There was virtually no difference in the two groups. Most of the participants of the study had returned to their natural state of happiness, whether they had been generally happy or generally unhappy people before the life-changing events of winning the lottery or losing the use of limbs. Both groups had largely adjusted to their new circumstances, despite the drastic circumstantial changes that they had experienced, and also despite the drastically different circumstances that each group was now in. As a whole, the paraplegics were just as happy and satisfied with their lives as the lottery winners were; what determined their happiness level six months after the event had nothing to do with the event and everything to do with how happy they had been beforehand.[13] If that's not the clearest indicator that happiness is not dictated by external factors, I don't know what is! And the reason for it is psychological adaptation.

I've seen this happen firsthand. My doubles partner from our high school tennis team was in a tragic car accident and became a paraplegic. At one point he became suicidal. But as time passed, he told anyone who would listen that becoming a paraplegic was actually the best thing that ever happened to him, because it forced him to look internally rather than externally. He later wrote a book about his experience.

Psychological adaptation is one of the incredible feats of human design. When you are able to find a reasonable internal balance, you can recover internally and truly be "okay" in almost any situation. Of course, we all know many people who don't bounce back. Why? In my experience, psychological adaptation doesn't work when your natural state is one of fear or fight-or-flight, if you have too many memories wrongly labeled as "life or death."

The good news is that it is possible to change the labels on those memories, and therefore restore the internal balance that you need for psychological adaptation to work for you regardless of your circumstances. As you'll see in part 2, memory engineering can heal those memories and allow psychological adaptation to kick in again, the way it was designed to.

WE ARE WIRED FOR LOVING RELATIONSHIPS

After all this discussion of the body's natural mechanisms for happiness, you may be wondering: if we're built to be happy, why aren't we?

We are wired for love, but we are also wired for loving, kind relationships. George Vaillant, MD, director of Harvard University's Grant Study of Human Development, the "longest-running longitudinal studies of human development in history," summed up its findings like this: "The seventy-five years and twenty million dollars expended on the Grant Study points to a straightforward five-word conclusion: Happiness equals love. Full stop."[14] Love, in this context, is referring to loving relationships.

Loving relationships also have a direct impact on our health. According to a study reported in *USA Today*, if we have loving relationships, we are 300 percent more likely to be healthy than those in conflicted relationships. The converse is also true: if we have conflicted relationships, we are 300 percent more likely to contract illness and disease, and even die sooner, than those in loving relationships.[15] To say it another way, this love problem is literally killing us.

What's happening beneath those numbers? Well, a number of things. Too often, and also too often without malice, we find ourselves in relationships with people who are not able or willing to face us with the pure love that we deserve. There's an old saying that I think explains why we aren't all living in a love-based state: Hurt people hurt people. When we are exposed too often to people whose actions cause us pain or trauma, even without their intending to have that effect, our heart pulls the fire alarm: we are kicked out of our default, wired-for-love, positive setting and into the fear response, which, as we saw earlier, affects not just our mind but our bodies as well. This becomes the way that we approach the world, which both reinforces the behavior in our own lives and also passes it along to those we interact with.

This is especially true during our first years of life, as shown by the famous still face experiments.[16] In these experiments by Edward Tronick, PhD, a baby sits across from her mother. First, the mother shows great enthusiasm for the baby and responds positively to everything the baby does—and the baby responds very positively, too. Then the mother turns away for a moment. When she turns back to the baby, she has a completely blank expression. The baby tries to reach out to the mother and yells to get a response from her, and when the mother remains completely nonresponsive, the baby very quickly gets agitated and upset.

We're the same way as we age, too. Just as a superficial example: if a stranger sits next to you on the plane, how do you feel if they never make eye contact with you or say hello for the entire trip? How do you feel when they look you in the eye, smile, and introduce themselves? Even if they go right back to their book or phone for the entire trip, doesn't that make the experience feel completely different?

Relationships are what give our experiences, and our memories, meaning. Outside of circumstantial danger, relationship issues truly are issues of life and death, even though we rarely treat them that way.

The Two Laws

Aligning perfectly with the two different stages of brain waves (before beta and after beta), we also have two "laws" preprogrammed in our heart, and they're almost polar opposites. But they are both there for a reason and have important jobs.

The first is the Law of Externals. The Law of Externals says that outside factors are the most important things in life, beginning with physical survival extending all the way to whatever externals make our physical lives more comfortable and pleasurable. The Law of Externals says that we need physical things to survive and thrive— that happiness comes from our stuff, our job titles, our money, and power over others. It leads people to demand "what I want when I want it."

The priority is to get the end results that benefit you the most, even if that means others have to lose or get hurt. The Law of Externals prioritizes your own needs over others and self-protection over relationships. It's living a life of seeking pleasure and avoiding pain. The governing motive is *self-interest*.

Every mechanism inside us has a positive function, including the Law of Externals. Until sometime between ages six and twelve, children primarily operate according to this law. Survival truly is at stake, often many times a day.

However, when our conscious mind develops, sometime between the ages of six and twelve, we're supposed to shift to the second law programmed in our heart, which is the Law of Internals.

The Law of Internals says that maintaining an internal state of love, joy, and peace, as opposed to fear, is the most important thing, regardless of external circumstances. It results in doing what's right simply because it's the right thing to do, regardless of whether it benefits you in the short term or even causes you pain. It means prioritizing a positive process over profitable product, although often when everyone is feeling good and supported, the results show that you can have both at the same time. The Law of Internals says that happiness comes from within, from doing good in the world and putting good into the lives of everyone you interact with. The governing motive is *love*.

The Law of Internals is hardwired to our *conscience*, or what I like to think of as our "love compass"; it's the part of us that tells us the best course of action based on the lens of love and activates our ability to do it through our beliefs, thoughts, feelings, brain chemistry, and actions. In other words, this law is about doing what is right and best for all parties involved, right now, whether it results in personal pain, pleasure, or neither.

One modern thought leader in the self-help world teaches that "the secret of life is self-interest." This may seem accurate, but the truth is that self-interest is only the secret to death.

Remember how our brain chemistry works: self-interest is rooted in our survival instinct, which is rooted in fear, which leads to all the negative results in the list above.

The Law of Externals insists on only one winner: me. With this guiding me, I might not go out of my way to prevent others from winning and may even be happy to see others win—as long as there is no question that I am getting exactly what I want in the exact quantity that I want. If I'm not, then my care for others may be out the window, at least until I can get back in my comfort zone. If everyone lived according to the Law of Internals, it would solve so many of the crippling social problems that plague us today. I believe that many of our worst problems are rooted in the system of selfishness. And of course, the greatest irony is that, according to the Harvard Grant study, experiencing an internal state of love is the only thing that will truly satisfy you long term—not the material and superficial things the Law of Externals prioritizes.

The Law of Internals is designed to guide you to win-win-win situations for all parties involved to the best of your ability:

The first win is for other people directly involved.

The second win is for all peripheral people who might be affected.

The third win is for you.

That's right, your win is the last one, not the first or second. You don't win until you make sure others win. The Law of Internals means escaping the cycle of avoiding pain and pursuing pleasure to say, "Dadgummit, I'm going to do what's right, what's moral, and what's best for the larger community." Everyone benefits, but you do it because you're living first for the good of others, and then for yourself.

Humans are wired to have relationships. The Law of Externals tends to be about my external circumstances and relationship with myself, or others who have influence over whether I get what I want or not. The Law of Internals is about *all* relationships—including those with myself, those I know, and even those I don't know about.

Now, you've got to put the Law of Internals on pause if you're in life-threatening crisis. If you're in crisis, you do need to take care of yourself, or you won't be able to find a win-win-win. In fact, putting yourself first when you are in a crisis is often the most loving thing to do for others, because you're equipping yourself to help others more in the long run. But if you're not in crisis, then the first two wins are for other people, and you don't get your win unless others win.

How do children naturally switch from the Law of Externals to the Law of Internals? Remember, we have the Law of Internals preprogrammed in our heart, just like the Law of Externals. When we're in the delta-theta brainwave state, although we do have a conscience, we're primarily operating according to the Law of Externals, with our brainwave state protecting us from the stressful effects of fear. At the same time, ideally, our parents are operating according to the Law of Internals and are pouring love into us—ten positive experiences to one negative. We receive clear consequences when we do something wrong or harmful, but they're given in love, not anger or harshness.

If the Law of Internals is modeled consistently for us as children, we're able to successfully shift naturally to this law at some point on our way into adulthood. We don't need to be taught; we will naturally transition spiritually and mentally toward valuing a win-win-win over just a personal win, and prioritizing the internal.

However, if we haven't been treated according to the Law of Internals, or if we've had role models that don't exhibit it as a trait on a regular basis, we hit a crossroads— a divergence in the path that leads us either to the Law of Externals to govern our decision-making or to the Law of Internals. These two laws lead to very different ways of life: one leads to happiness no matter what our circumstances, while one leads straight to constant insecurity no matter what our resources. We'll learn more about both of these paths in chapter 4.

To summarize: the human body was designed to work well, even miraculously, if all its mechanisms are functioning properly, just like a car or a boat or a computer or any other complex system. One of my friends is a medical doctor and genetics researcher, and he tells me that if the human body operates largely without stress (the way it should), it is designed to live and remain predominantly healthy for about 120 years. That goes for you, for me, for your cousin Billy, for the woman in the checkout line, for the guy you pass on the highway: everybody is designed to make it to 120 and healthy.

If we were functioning the way we were built to function, thanks to all of these features built into the human design, our thoughts, feelings, and beliefs would consist of love, joy, and peace for the great majority of our time. Regardless of what happened, we would have a basic belief in ourself as a good person—no better or worse than anybody else, but still very good. We'd be able to easily access the rule of love in our conscience, know how to create kind and loving relationships, and make win-win-win decisions. Whenever we would do something wrong, we would say, "I'm sorry," confess it to clear the air, make whatever amends might be called for, and start again.

When we'd experience pain in our lives—and we all would—we might be disappointed, hurt, or grieving, but not overwhelmed by stress or despair. If we were ever in a truly life-threatening situation, our hypothalamus would switch on our life-or-death survival response, which would take over just until the danger passed, and then because of psychological adaptation, we'd be back to our normal state of love, joy, and peace. And we'd live about 120 years, primarily healthy.

This is what I've learned over the past thirty-plus years

of working with clients; it's validated by science, and for the most part it's old news. When our bodies, minds, and spirits operate in harmony with one another, and the way they were designed to work, it's beautiful. Even miraculous.

WHEN PAIN IS NO LONGER A PROBLEM

I need to clarify one important point, however. When I say our default setting is positive, I'm not talking about a pain-free life.

Today, pain management is a 635 billion-dollar industry, and it seems to be growing.[17] Why? Pain demands a response.

Much of that pain comes from the illusions created by your memories, which we can heal together in this book. I want to say that there is a path toward "the perfect life for you," but I'm going to stop short of that, because if I use the word "perfect," I'm concerned you'll get the impression that I mean a life with no health problems or pain ever, and that is not what I mean at all. There is pain for you, there is pain for me, there was pain for Abraham Lincoln, there is pain for the movie stars, there is pain for everybody. Pain is not an accident, it's not a flaw, and it's not a mistake. It doesn't necessarily mean anything's wrong. Sometimes it's a passage to the next level of your life. Rather than "your perfect life," what exists is your best possible life, experiencing love, joy, and peace through the pain, not necessarily without the pain. For what it's worth, your physical and external circumstances do typically get better, and often beyond your imagination. Why? Because you aren't malfunctioning anymore.

I was told many years ago that Freud said, "Idealism is the cause of all human suffering." I'm no fan of Freud, but I think he's absolutely right about that. Idealism is *comparison* and *expectation* put together. Idealism results from an external end result goal and comparing yourself to other people, and on the basis of that comparison, needing a certain outcome to be okay. We'll talk more about this in chapter 4 as well.

The best thing for your future is not necessarily what you think it is now. I've worked with a number of very wealthy and famous people over the last twenty years. One in ten are rich and happy—the other nine are rich and full of anxiety and stress. And these are people about whom most of us think, *If I only had what they had, I would be really happy.* Expecting that your life has to be a certain way will kill you, but even more than that, those expectations of what a good life looks like are almost always wrong. For that one in ten, being a famous, rich musician probably is the best life for them, but those other nine might have been better off being a lawyer or an accountant—or even just dealing with life in a better way internally. Or maybe best yet, still being rich and famous but living in love rather than fear. The one common thing I have found with the one in ten is that they don't really care about money or fame very much. They just love the music.

For most of us, finding our perfect life is a journey, and we don't end up where we thought we would.

The question is, are you on the path of your best life, or are you on the path of fear, anxiety, and stress?

Both paths have pain. But on one path, everything painful can be meaningful, like the pain of giving birth. On the other path, pain turns into festering sores and infections, and worst of all is meaningless.

Think about your last bad day again, and what made it a bad day. Maybe you experienced the worst physical pain of your life, or the worst emotional pain in a relationship. Maybe you weren't accepted to the college you really wanted to go to or you didn't receive the promotion you thought would allow you to do what you most wanted. Maybe someone hurt you. Or very often, nothing may be terribly wrong; you just want things that you don't have.

What if, without altering the actual events, you could change it from a bad day to a good day, or at least to an okay day? What would it be worth to have almost all the bad days for the rest of your life not be bad days?

I'm not talking about some pie in the sky, "a million dollars is on the way to me right now" kind of affirmation that your unconscious doesn't believe. I'm talking about an automatic, default, truthful, effortless response of, "That's not a big deal. I'm fine!" or "That hurt like heck, but I'm going to be okay!"

Does that mean you don't experience pain? Nope, the pain's still there.

Does it mean that the person who was mean and ugly to you was now nice to you? No, they were still mean and ugly.

Does that mean you somehow got into that college or got that job? No, that didn't happen, either.

Does it mean you are now rich or famous? Nope.

Does it mean if you are rich and famous that you are guaranteed another hit song or movie? No way.

It means that, in spite of that painful thing, you are still internally experiencing thoughts and feelings of love, joy, peace, and positive self-worth. It means you think, "Yes, this hurts, but it's not a bad day. I'm still okay." Or it is one of those rare catastrophically painful events where you do, and should feel crushed, but you also know you will bounce back and be okay, and you do. The biggest change will be when the "get through it with stress" day is now a great day—and the circumstances are unchanged!

Pain is no longer a problem; in fact, it's now a gateway to growth and greater meaning and purpose in your life, which leads to even greater experiences.

The belief that pleasure is always positive and pain is always negative is simply false. Very often pain is the best thing that could happen to us, and the wrong kind of pleasure will destroy us.

Let me promise you this: when you can learn to disconnect pain from fear, when you can experience physical pain without being triggered into distress or panic, your life is going to feel like a walk in the park. I guarantee it.

If we work the way we were designed to work, our default experience should be positive—physically, mentally, and spiritually. However, blockages, breakages, and shortages can dramatically impact whether we actually experience that default. Our heart was made to pump blood efficiently throughout our bodies—when it doesn't, we call it a malfunction. Our muscles were made to move us around easily—when they don't, we call it a malfunction. Our immune system was made to recognize threats to our health and destroy them on a cellular level—when it doesn't, or when it overreacts to a non-threatening entity, we call it a malfunction.

It is time to acknowledge that the same is true for our mental processes. Our hypothalamus was made to switch on our stress response when we're in a life-threatening situation only[18]—*when it switches it on when our lives aren't in danger, there's a malfunction.*

I believe the source of that malfunction is in our memories.

So let's take a deeper look at how we make memories in the first place.

CHAPTER TWO

Making Memories

It may be hard to believe that memories are the source of your biggest problem. How can your performance at work, your health issues, or your relationship issues today be the result of your memories of events long ago?

According to memory researcher Julia Shaw, PhD, "When we define ourselves (You-ness) we may think about our gender, ethnicity, age, occupation, markers of what we have achieved like education, buying a house, getting married, having children or reaching retirement. We may also think about personality characteristics— whether we tend to be optimistic or pessimistic, funny or serious, selfish or selfless. On top of this we likely think about how we compare to others. However, while all these descriptors may be more or less appropriate ways of defining who you are, the true root of your 'you-ness' almost certainly lies in your personal memories."[1]

If memories define who we are and are the source of why we're malfunctioning, it's worth taking a deeper look at how they work.

Although the field of psychology has always known that our current issues go back to our memories, the scientific study of memories is relatively new. In this chapter, I'd like to share with you my own theory of how memories work, based on thirty years of client work, personal study and research, my own experience, and the supporting science.

What Julia Shaw calls personal memories I would call source memories. They're the images we store in our heart, they're subject to errors that can affect our whole life (as you'll see below), and they can be healed by the memory engineering process you'll learn later.

I believe these source memories come from three primary areas: personal experience, imagination, and past generations.

MEMORIES FROM OUR PERSONAL EXPERIENCE

Several years ago I visited the Grand Canyon with my family. As we all walked up to the observation point and took it in for the first time, here's what I remember. First, I took in data from my five senses: I saw the colors and depth of the canyon, I heard a hawk cry and the footsteps of my family, I felt a cool breeze on my arms, etc. Then, internally, I felt awe and amazement. Next, I thought, Wow, it looks different in person. Finally, I acted by saying what I was thinking: "Wow, it looks different in person!"

That memory seems pretty straightforward, doesn't it? That's how all of us experience our lives on a daily basis: we see (i.e., experience with our five senses), feel, think, and then act. Our memories are formed from what we "see" with our five senses.

Many of us believe our memories of our personal experiences are like a video recording of the world around us. We experience something with our five senses, we record an accurate account of what happened in the form of a memory, and when we remember that experience, we see exactly what happened. But according to the latest research, that's not remotely how memories are made. In fact, many researchers today say that it is actually more accurate to refer to our memories, even of our own experiences, as illusions.

Why? What you're *seeing* is not just objective data from your five senses. Everything you see with your physical eyes (and experience with all your other senses) is first filtered through the lens of your already existing memories.

So how *do* we see? To use the computer analogy again, we come out of the box preprogrammed. The majority of us are born into bodies that know how to breathe and to communicate enough to get food and care. We also come preloaded with cellular memories, but we'll talk more about these later in this chapter.

Then, once we're born and start experiencing the world for ourselves, data enters through our senses at literally the speed of light—186,000 miles per second. This data does not come in like a video, but as electrical and chemical impulses, which are both run first through our *already existing* memories that probably number in the trillions. (The latest findings say our brain's memory capacity is about one quadrillion bytes, or pretty much the size of the entire Internet.[2]) Any previous memories that have data even vaguely similar to the current circumstance—especially life-threatening ones, as we'll see below—are prioritized.

Once those impulses are filtered through all those memories, the unconscious mind assembles all that data and creates a finished internal picture or video, and that's our new memory. That's what we "see," which leads to our feelings, thoughts, body chemistry, and actions. Our memories are a lot more like Photoshop files than video recordings. All of this happens virtually instantaneously, automatically, and continually.

What this means is that the resulting video or picture (what we would call our memory) is frequently not exactly what happened. In fact, it could be anywhere from 1 percent to 99 percent different.

To give you an example, let's take a deeper look at my experience of the Grand Canyon. My previous memories (internal images) of the Grand Canyon were the pictures I had seen in National Geographic and maybe some other imagined images of what I thought the Grand Canyon might be like, based on those magazine pictures and what others had told me. Those images formed the lens through which I took in the sensory data of the real Grand Canyon. Since I had only experienced similar data in the form of magazine pictures and my imagination based on those pictures, the real-life data far exceeded and was infinitely more beautiful and awe-inspiring than my pre-existing internal pictures, so my emotional response was one of beauty and awe, and my resulting thoughts, body chemistry, and actions aligned with that response.

My family and I were recently talking about visiting the Grand Canyon, and my son Harry said, "My memory of the Grand Canyon is throwing up!" I had forgotten that we had taken a helicopter ride during that trip and Harry got airsick. We all were exposed to the same sensory data—seeing the canyon, hearing the sounds, taking the helicopter ride. But while the primary memory of the Grand Canyon was beauty and awe for three of us, for Harry it was very different!

In his book *Enlightenment Now*, Steven Pinker explains the well-researched phenomenon called the *availability heuristic*, sometimes called the *availability bias*. It means that the more easily a fact or situation comes to mind, the more likely we believe it's going to happen.

"Frequent events leave stronger memory traces, so stronger memories generally indicate more-frequent events.... But whenever a memory turns up high in the result list of the mind's search engine for reasons other than frequency— because it is recent, vivid, gory, distinctive, or upsetting— people will overestimate how likely it is in the world."

For example, Pinker notes that more people are afraid of flying than driving, even though statistically death by car crash is far more likely than death by plane crash, because plane crashes are reported more often in the media. That's the availability bias at work.[3]

What determines the availability of our memories is how vivid they are, which is determined by several factors.

The Fear Factor

Let's take the Grand Canyon example one step further. What if I had first visited the Grand Canyon on a school trip, and I witnessed a scary accident: someone from my class was leaning against the barrier, the barrier broke, and that person fell and broke his leg?

My experience visiting the Grand Canyon with my family as an adult would be very different, wouldn't it? The data coming in through my five senses might be the same, but what I thought I saw would change. For instance, in the first scenario, I don't have a clear memory of whether my wife or sons were approaching or leaning against the barrier. (I don't even remember Harry getting airsick on the helicopter!) I was focused on the canyon itself, because I had no reason not to be.

But in the second scenario, I may see my younger son running toward the barrier recklessly, when perhaps another observer would say he was simply walking fast and was nowhere close to the edge.

Where the sensory data made me feel awe in the first scenario, I would likely feel terrified in the second. I would think of my friend falling off the ledge, and as a result yell out, "Get away from that barrier!," run toward my son, and probably grab his arm and yank him back.

Whenever we experience the emotion of fear, our body is flooded with adrenaline, cortisol, and a host of other fight-or-flight chemicals. This is commonly known as the fear response or the stress response, and what this book has been calling the "life-or-death" response, because as we saw that was its original purpose: to physically save our life.

The biological life-or-death response has been shown to make the memory more vivid and powerful.[4] The more fear (and adrenaline) you experience during a certain event, the more vivid it will be, and the more likely to become your lens for similar circumstances in the future.

In fact, negative memories in general tend to be more vivid because of what's known as the *negativity bias*. "Bad things loom larger in our minds than good things," says author and brain scientist Jeff Stibel. "We evolved that way because paying attention to potential dangers is necessary for survival."[5] That's why Harry remembered throwing up more than the beauty of the canyon.

However, "more vivid" or "more powerful" doesn't necessarily mean "more accurate." In *The Memory Illusion*, memory researcher Dr. Julia Shaw details many other ways errors and misconceptions can be introduced to our memories, and how often we can be sure we remember something that in fact never happened, or at least we never witnessed.

According to Shaw, Thomas Schilling and his colleagues at University of Trier in Germany published a study in 2013 on how stress impacts memory. They found that the release of cortisol makes memory stronger but also more susceptible to errors. She uses witnessing a bank robbery as an example: you're likely to clearly remember the gun pointed at you, but unlikely to remember other important details, like the face of the person holding the gun.[6]

To make matters worse, trauma memories tend to get worse over time, unlike other memories, to the point that people remember experiencing more trauma than they actually did. In one study, researchers asked Desert Storm veterans about specific events during their time of service at two different times: one month after returning and then two years after returning. The results showed that 88 percent changed at least one answer, and 61 percent changed more than one—with most remembering more negative events than the first time.[7]

That's why many researchers say what we call our memories are really more like illusions.[8] And it's why four people witness the same crime, but when FBI detectives interview each of them afterward, they all say they saw something a little bit different. Of course, they saw some common things too, but the detectives know that each person will report seeing something slightly different. In fact, if all four people have exactly the same story and words about an unsolved crime, the detectives (who apparently know a little more about memory errors than most of us) automatically suspect someone's lying.

Early Childhood

In addition to our negative memories, the memories we make in early childhood are also prioritized above those made later in life (even if we don't remember them consciously), because those are typically accompanied by more adrenaline and little if any rational editing. When have we ever experienced anything as strongly as when we were children? As we discussed in chapter 1, up to the age of roughly six to twelve, we are primarily in the delta-theta brainwave state, which means most of our experiences instantly become source memories, whether we're interpreting what's happening accurately or not.

You can probably already imagine how many errors get deeply programmed into us during early childhood and how often we experience events as traumatic as children when, if experienced as adults, they would have little to no effect on us. I call these "Popsicle memories," and we'll talk much more about them in the next chapter.

MEMORIES FROM OUR IMAGINATION

In addition to our personal experience, we also create source memories from our imagination. Our imagination—or what I call our *image maker*—can create memories that are just as powerful as our personal experience. Remember the second German definition of the word "imagination" is to create.

I'll give you an example. When my son Harry was little, one of his favorite things in the world to do was swim. Harry was the kid who, when he was around two or three years old, would jump in the water in full clothes whenever he saw a swimming pool, lake, or ocean. One time we were at the Opryland Hotel to see the Christmas lights, and he did that in the middle of winter. My wife, Hope, had to jump in after him in all her clothes.

That is, until Harry saw the movie *Jaws*. We had a trip to the lake that had been planned for a while the weekend after he'd seen the movie. Now, all of a sudden, he didn't want to go at all, and when we got there, he would not go anywhere near the water. He was obviously in physical stress: his face was red, and he was visibly agitated and upset.

Nothing had changed about the water. Nothing had changed about Harry's experience in the water. He'd always had a great time! The only thing that had changed was that he now had a memory based on the movie he had seen telling him, "The water will kill you. There's going to be blood everywhere. You're going to be ripped open, you're going to be screaming, and it's going to be horrible."

Harry never connected his new fear of the water to the movie *Jaws*. In fact, he tried to rationalize that it was simply that he now knew the water was unsafe—which, to our knowledge, he had never thought before he saw the movie.

That memory completely changed his meaning of what the water meant to him. Just thinking about the water immediately affected his physiology, chemistry, and behavior.

You can probably think of a similar example in your own life. Memories from movies and our own image maker can be just as powerful as anything we experience.

Recent research has also shown that simply imagining an event can create a false memory that affects people as powerfully as if it were true.[9] A famous example is the "spilling the punchbowl" experiment, conducted by memory researchers Ira Hyman and Joel Pentland at Western Washington University. Participants were asked how well they could remember experiences from their early childhood, which they were told had been provided by their parents.

The researchers gave the participants general information about each event and then asked them to vividly imagine the event and tell the researchers what they saw in detail. Most of these events had actually happened, except one: an incident where they had spilled the punchbowl at a family friend's wedding when they were five.

After three visits, a week apart, the study found that 25 percent of the participants created a psychologically verified false memory of spilling the punchbowl.

As Julia Shaw puts it, "This demonstrates that we can misattribute the source of our childhood memories, thinking that something we imagined actually happened, internalizing information that someone suggested to us and spinning it into a part of our personal past. It is an extreme form of confabulation that can be induced by someone else by engaging your imagination."[10]

In the 1970s and 1980s, counseling clients began remembering all kinds of abuse they had never remembered before.

This was a time when psychologists were becoming more aware of the reality of child sexual abuse, and well-meaning therapists would sometimes ask repeatedly, "Are you *sure* no one ever touched you inappropriately when you were a child? You have all the symptoms, and it would explain everything." The client's mind quite naturally begins imagining what such a scenario would be like, and voilà— all of a sudden that client begins vividly remembering instances of abuse. Some of these memories were real and provided important breakthroughs to allow healing. But in many instances, it was later proven that people were "recovering" memories that had actually been created by their imagination, prompted by the therapists' questions.

MEMORIES FROM PAST GENERATIONS

The final, and one of the most fascinating, areas of memory is a phenomenon that we are only beginning to understand. Just in the last few years, research has shown that memories, especially trauma memories, can actually be passed down from generation to generation through both nature (genetically) and nurture (absorbing or learning memories from our parents or childhood environment).

Beginning with the nurture aspect, we can all probably think of examples of learning to fear certain events because we see that our parents do. Groundbreaking research by Rachel Yeshuda, PhD, has substantiated what many of us have guessed to be true. Her studies have shown that descendants of Holocaust survivors have altered stress hormones, making them more prone to anxiety disorders, PTSD, and obesity, among other risks.[11] The traumatic memories, and their symptoms, had been passed down in some way to the next generation.

How might this have happened? Additional studies with rats suggest that mothers transmit a particular smell that transmits specific fear memories. The lateral amygdala is the specific part of the brain that receives the "smell-transmitted fear," according to researchers, and infants can receive this information very early from their mothers, even about events that happened during the mother's pregnancy. The lead researcher, Jacek Debiec, MD, PhD, of the University of Michigan, said, "These maternally transmitted memories are long-lived, whereas other types of infant learning, if not repeated, rapidly perish."[12]

In addition to the nurture component, research is also showing that there's a nature component of inheriting memories. Researchers at Emory University discovered that traumatic experiences can be genetically passed down in mice through the DNA.[13] Further studies on mice showed how the DNA receives information about the father's trauma: specific cells excrete a type of "extracellular vesicle" that attaches to the sperm and transfers information about any traumatic memories the father has. By using in vitro fertilization, the study showed that the offspring didn't have to have any physical contact with the father to receive his trauma memories.[14]

Although similar research is just beginning to look at the effect of stress on human sperm, this research implies that we might experience trauma symptoms from events that didn't happen to us, even if we never had personal contact with the previous generation they did happen to.

New research in this area is coming out all the time. For example, in 2019, researchers at Tel Aviv University discovered that RNA molecules can send instructions for adaptation or malfunction to future generations and that these signals can influence a number of different physiological processes. It's yet another way the experiences of past generations can be passed down biologically. According to the *Jerusalem Post*, "the findings, [lead researcher Oded] Rechavi said, contradict one of the most basic dogmas in modern biology, where it has long been thought that brain activity could have no impact at all on the fate of future generations."[15]

We don't yet know how to recognize or distinguish these genetic trauma memories, but based on this research, we're likely to have them. And if we do have them, they're extremely unlikely to fade over time, because we also know that trauma memories are more protected than other memories.

Years ago, my good friend and colleague Doris Rapp,

MD, the recognized worldwide pioneer of children's environmental medicine, shared a concept with me I use all the time. When it comes to how we deal with stress, she says it's like everyone has a "stress barrel." Once it's full, even the smallest stress can be a trigger for a massive reaction. The key is keeping your stress barrel as empty as possible.

It's safe to say that these inherited trauma memories are certainly filling up at least part of our stress barrels, even though we don't know what these specific memories are. It takes a lot of energy from your mind and immune system to keep those memories protected and repressed—energy that could be used for a more productive day, expressing positive emotions, or balancing brain chemistry, for example.

THE INTERPRETATION IS PART OF THE MEMORY

In addition to our memory of the event, which itself can be skewed, our interpretation of the event is another component that influences the memory.

Here's how I often explain it to my clients: Think of your memories as being organized like a filing system. Every memory has a label or marker on it, much like a label on a file folder. No memory is floating out there on its own; every memory is associated with a label. On your computer, you might have files with labels like Utilities, Groceries, or Maintenance. You can easily go to the file folder labeled Utilities and pull up all your utilities files. Every file is somewhere; whether it's organized specifically, like "Utilities, May 2015" or more generally, like a document just sitting on your computer desktop.

If you're on the computer, which is similar to how your brain works, you can do a custom search for all files to have the computer pull up everything that's associated with a specific word or phrase.

The difference is that your mind's labels aren't Utilities or Groceries or Maintenance; they're things like Anger, Forgiveness, Self-Worth, Identity, Safe, and Life or Death. These labels represent the interpretation you've given to your memories.

Memories can also have more than one label assigned to them: the same memory might be in the Life or Death folder and the Mother folder.

Unlike computer files, however, every memory is also encoded according to how fear-based or love-based the memory is. You can think of it as a rating on a continuum of negative 10 to positive 10, where negative 10 is 100 percent fear-based, and positive 10 is 100 percent love-based.

Your mind uses this rating to prioritize the memory. The top priority goes to Life or Death–related meanings, while labels like Self-Worth or Helping Others would be a good ways down your priority list, and typically not on the list at all if a Life or Death–labeled file is currently active.

Negative labels have a negative scale; positive labels have a positive scale. Remember the still face experiment. If you do something and someone smiles at you, that's positive feedback, and it ends up in a positive file folder with a positive rating. When you think back on that positive memory, you will tend to feel and think something positive (similar thoughts and feelings to those you felt during the original event), thus creating a new positive memory of your current experience. And you will tend to feel positive about doing or experiencing similar things again in the future.

If you do something and someone frowns or scolds you, that's negative feedback, and it will get put into a negative file folder with a negative rating, which depends on how much adrenaline was released at the time of the original event. If the event has a negative rating, you will tend to feel negative, create a new negative memory, and likely resist doing a similar thing again.

These labels allow your unconscious mind to filter through everything that has ever happened to you, plus everything passed down from your ancestry, in a nanosecond. They form your belief system and worldview—in other words, your memories are why you have the opinions you do. You may be open to changing your opinion if presented with the right facts by the right person, but only if your opinions are not tied to any fear or danger memories. If they are, you will resist changing that belief, almost to the death.

We can see this clearly in the increasingly polarized political climate in the United States, where each side accuses the other of reporting "fake news." How is it that each side believes "facts" that seem to be the polar opposite of what the other group believes? Political science researcher Dan Kahan, JD, at Yale dug into the specific issue of climate change, and he and his colleagues found that those with the highest "science literacy and technical reasoning capacity" were not the most likely to agree on a certain statement about climate change, but were simply the most likely to be "culturally polarized." In other words, the smarter you are, the more likely you are to use your intellect to find reasons the group you're already a part of is right—regardless of what is actually true![16]

Similarly, researchers Brendan Nyhan, PhD, and Jason Reifler, PhD, ran a series of experiments in which participants read either an article with a misleading claim from a politician or an article with that misleading claim and a correction of that claim. According to the study, "results indicate that corrections frequently fail to reduce misperceptions among the targeted ideological group. We also document several instances of a 'backfire effect' in which corrections actually *increase* misperceptions among the group in question."[17]

I would say our memories are the source of why we do this: we have a fear memory associated with being accepted or rejected by a certain group, and belonging to that group, according to our memories, is an issue of life or death.

This is often how we discover ourselves liking some things and disliking others, like Republican or Democrat, beaches or mountains. We develop reasoning that appears logical, as long as those facts agree with our memories' labels and ratings. It happens in day-to-day situations, too. For example, if I'm six years old and my mother yells at me for spilling my grape juice on the new white carpet, I may have a 90 percent fear-based memory related to spilling something. In other words, that memory of spilling something goes into the Life or Death file, and it's rated at negative 9. I'm now strongly programmed to be afraid of spilling something. Now, for the rest of my life, I get a little stressed if I'm in a situation where something might spill (by me or someone else). If I do spill, I will likely feel some degree of anger, guilt, blame, or shame. So not spilling will cause me to feel better about myself, and I'm going to scrutinize my behavior for potential spilling situations—I'll be thinking about spilling inordinately often. How warped is that? My self-worth hanging on something everyone does from time to time that has nothing to do with a successful life.

I'll also probably be very critical of others when they spill something. I may have all sorts of rational reasons why I hate it so much when people spill drinks: *It's so inconsiderate. Now I have to take the time to clean up the mess. It's just a pet peeve of mine.* But the real reason is that it has a highly negative fear label associated with it and has nothing to do with any rational reason I may have come up with.

On the other hand, if my mother is kind and understanding when I make a mess (even if she administers loving discipline), I now have a 90 percent love-based memory about spilling something. That memory of spilling something might be filed in the Unconditional Love file, perhaps at a positive 9—and now I am strongly programmed not to be afraid of spilling something. And you have probably already guessed I am now far less likely to spill something.

This is a great example of how relationships give meaning to memories. What was the difference between the negative, positive, and neutral memories? In every instance, the grape juice ended up on the white carpet, and someone still had to clean it up. The difference was the way I experienced my *relationship* with my mom before and during that incident, which was based on her verbal and nonverbal reaction.

It's also a great example of how powerful our childhood

memories are. When we're in the delta-theta brainwave state as children, our memories are instantly programmed and prioritized in our subconscious—and our fear memories most of all. Consider why your mother may have reacted the way she did: Was she having a good day or a bad day? Was she reacting based on her own memory of spilling when she was a little girl, or the current circumstances? Regardless of the reason, this single moment is likely to impact your current and future relationships in many important ways.

OUR MEMORIES ARE MORE LIKE ILLUSIONS

Understanding that our memories are more like illusions than video recordings means we can be a lot less judgmental toward others and ourselves. If you find yourself judging someone else or getting angry, you can train yourself to think, "Okay, wait a minute. I don't need to leap to conclusions here, because that person may not have really said what I remember her saying, or meant it the way I am taking it. Let me suspend judgment and get some more information about how this was intended."

If you tend to judge yourself harshly, remember that you have generations of memories governing how you see the world, and those are what ultimately create your beliefs, thoughts, feelings, brain chemistry, and actions. We all do. I have no idea what unconscious or generational issues caused me to act like an arrogant, self-gratifying idiot for the first several years of my marriage. I have theories, but I certainly don't have evidence beyond a reasonable doubt. The best we can do is learn about the way we work, have compassion for ourselves and others, heal what we can heal no matter how long it takes, and be committed to living in the present moment in truth and love, from now on.

You may be thinking, "I'm not stressed—I'm doing fine." If so, you might be one of the rare few people who really are doing fine. If so, you probably don't need this book, and feel free to share it with someone who does.

But I have found that stress has become such a constant that most people don't even recognize it anymore unless they experience an extreme spike. As part of my own three-year study on the Healing Codes and other healing techniques, I found that more than 90 percent of those who tested as clinically stressed, based on a heart-rate variability test, said they weren't stressed.

As I said in the previous chapter, I don't believe this constant stress is a fatal flaw in our design as humans. I believe it's the result of a monster malfunction.

How did this happen?

It certainly didn't happen all at once. It's been happening slowly, one memory at a time, since the beginning of time. Near as I can figure, there are three parts to this monster malfunction:

1. The devolution of memory
2. Choosing the wrong system of right and wrong, so we end up making decisions like five-year-olds rather than adults
3. Losing our ability to make positive change in our lives, even when we want to

It all starts with the devolution of memory.

CHAPTER THREE

The Devolution of Memory

My mother's parents came over to the United States from Germany in the early 1900s. Her father, after years of hard work, was able to buy a beautiful southern homestead, and my mother loved living there. Unfortunately, during the Depression, the bank suddenly required my grandfather to pay the entire remainder of the mortgage on that property all at once, which was $500. This would be illegal for the bank to do today, but it happened to many people at the time. He didn't have the money, so he lost the plantation and had to move into a normal-size house in a small town. It didn't seem to bother my grandfather too much, but it was traumatic for my mother—she was negatively affected by that event for the rest of her life.

Growing up, my dad told me a thousand times that Mom had a problem with money, meaning that she was paranoid about losing our house. She spent thirty-five years saying, "We can't go on vacation [or do many other things], we have to put money toward the house," because internally and unconsciously, she was afraid we would lose it.

In those moments, my mom was not the mature, smart, rational woman she usually was. She was, for the purposes of our discussion, a five-year-old again, complete with immaturity, irrationality, and tantrum-like panic.

When Hope and I were newly married, we had a pretty significant financial downturn. One night, as I was lying awake worrying, I felt something evil come over me and had this terrifying thought, clear as day: *If I lose this house, I'm going to die.*

Sure, losing our house would be hard. But it wasn't going to literally kill me. Where did that belief come from?

To understand where it came from, and how our default human experience went from positive to negative, we first need to look back at the way our memories evolved over millennia of human experience. In fact, I wouldn't call it evolution—I'd call it a *devolution!*

Now that you know our negative memories are largely prioritized as we experience our lives and create new memories, you can also probably begin to imagine how quickly fear dominates our experience as a species—and gets worse with every generation.

This devolution shows up in these four key areas: the meaning of life and death, our inherited genetic memories, our inherited learned memories, and the interpretations of our memories.

THE DEVOLUTION OF THE MEANING OF
LIFE AND DEATH

The first part of the devolution of memory happened in our definitions of life and death: both in our memories and eventually in our language.

As the story goes, the first man and the first woman lived in a garden, and they had only *one* memory that got the label of Life or Death: eating the fruit from a certain tree. We're also told they had zero problems. They had work to do that didn't seem to feel like onerous work to them. They were happy and healthy. They were naked, and it wasn't wrong to be naked; they had no guilt or inhibitions. In fact, *nothing* was wrong, except that one thing: eating the fruit from that one particular tree. That was the only matter of life or death, the only thing that would trigger their life-or-death response, the only thing that would stress them out, the only "temptation." In other words, it was the only thing associated with the words "kill" or "die."

Let's progress a little further into the prehistoric era, where now we have five to ten situations associated with the words "die" or "kill," such as predators, not finding enough food or water for the day, not finding shelter for the night, or someone with a bigger club.

Fast forward to the Middle Ages, when we faced the dangers of plagues and wars. In addition to all of the above, now a cough, or a weak king, or any number of situations that might precede sickness or war are memories with the Life or Death label. So now there are fifty to one hundred situations that mean "die" or "kill." And as we know from chapter 1, our brain is always going to prioritize any memory even *remotely* related to a life-or-death situation.

Today we have hundreds or even thousands of situations that our memories have labeled as Life or Death because of some trauma in the past. If your great-grandfather owed back taxes to the IRS that eventually caused him to lose his house, checking the mail may trigger the life-or-death response for you. If your parents often fought in ways that left your mother in tears, someone crying may trigger the life-or-death response for you.

You would probably not say any of those things were going to "kill" you. You just experience some stress when checking the mail, or you just feel anxiety when you see someone crying. No big deal. It's just one of your pet peeves or a personality trait.

But if you're experiencing any emotion based in fear, such as anger, frustration, irritation, resentment, bitterness, unforgiveness, extreme sadness without extreme loss, anxiety, or any other similar emotion, that means a related source memory, whether you realize it or not, has the Life or Death label; your heart is physiologically responding as if your life literally were in danger.

Remember what we said in chapter 1: we were created to only experience the life-or-death response (or the stress response, as we often call it today) if our lives are in physical danger. As a result of our programming always prioritizing fear memories, we have devolved to a place where almost anything could be related to a meaning of die or kill, trigger our life-or-death response, and initiate stress, negativity, and selfishness.

For example, have you ever said or thought something like, "It'll kill me to see my team lose this game," or "I've got to get home before the rain starts" or "These letters from the IRS are killing me," or " I'm going to hurt somebody if this problem doesn't get solved"?

I vividly remember as a teenager feeling like I was going to die if the Tennessee Vols football team lost their game on Saturday. And sure enough, Hope would tell me after we married that if Tennessee lost on Saturday, I didn't recover until about Thursday. I was sad, irritable, and spent most of the week looking forward to them winning on the following Saturday, even though they often didn't. What I know now is that Tennessee winning or losing a football game, to my heart, was directly connected to my sense of self-worth. How ridiculous is that? I have zero control over that event, and even if I did, it had little to do with the important issues of my life—my relationships, my job, my health, etc. I now know this belief was learned and embedded in my memories from my dad and older brother, who were my heroes.

Our language is both a symptom and a cause of the devolution. On one hand, if you find yourself saying or thinking, "This is killing me" or "I'm dying here" on a regular basis, it might be a sign that you actually do have a life-or-death memory triggered by your current circumstance. Of course, you don't mean it literally—but if you're experiencing any fear-based emotion, your heart does. The same is true if you find yourself feeling that way, even if you would never use those words.

To add fuel to the fire, our own words, or rather their deeper definitions and meaning, can affect the kind of label a memory receives, too. For most generations in history, the words "die" or "kill" meant one thing: physical death. Guess what: because of your heart's safety features, when it comes to killing and dying, it does not have a sense of humor.

If you haven't had your heart's safety measures released (we'll talk more about how to do that in part 2), and you say, think, or feel something like "I am dying here" or "This is killing me," your heart immediately sends out the guys with guns, as they did with me at the airport. It does not reason it out. It doesn't say, "Oh, yeah, he thought 'dying,' but he's only talking about a parking place." That is what your conscious mind does; your heart would rather be safe than sorry, so your heart pulls the fire alarm.

The problem, of course, is that having this overreaction time and again is physically and emotionally killing us—as we learned from Dr. Lipton's research on how cells get sick. Stress is the root cause of all illness and disease. It's why Andrew Weil, MD, says, "All illness is psychosomatic."[1] He doesn't mean you're imagining it; he means it's a result of stress, or what I'm calling the life-or-death response.

So try to catch yourself saying, thinking, or feeling, "This is killing me." Even when you think you don't mean it, you might just be right!

THE DEVOLUTION OF OUR INHERITED MEMORIES

The second part of the devolution has to do with our accumulating genetic trauma memories.

Do you have a memory of someone you love dearly being run over by a train?

Do you have a memory of someone dear to you being violently murdered in front of you?

Do you have a memory of your children being abused?

Do you have a memory of your parents abandoning you?

Do you have a memory of your brother dying of a rare illness when you were a child?

Maybe none of these things have ever happened to you—I certainly hope that they haven't. But chances are you've got shades of every one of those memories in your heart, even if these events never happened to you personally. It happened in your ancestry, and that impression is being passed down. These genetic memories are full of errors, yet they continue to accumulate in the stress barrels of each generation, taking energy that could be better spent on optimizing our health, our relationships, our careers, the lives of others, and the world we live in.

How would you feel if any of those events were happening right now? How would you feel if someone dear to you were being abused, harmed, or even murdered in front of your eyes?

That's what your heart is experiencing. It is surely a weaker fear than if it were actually happening now, because much less adrenaline is being produced, but you're still feeling the negativity. Everything stored in your heart is happening to you *right now* in 360-degree surround sound, 24/7. Your unconscious doesn't differentiate between past, present, and future, or between real and imagined. Your heart is treating those memories as your present-tense reality, even if your conscious mind has no idea they're there. So not only does your heart treat them as real, it treats them as if they're happening right now and uses them as a lens to read your current circumstances. You can imagine how you'd feel if you were in a life-threatening situation right now; it would be "all hands on deck," and everything else can wait.

When your heart goes "all hands on deck" over something that happened two hundred years ago in your ancestry, what gets put on hold is your digestion, blood sugar balancing, immune function, creativity, the ability to truly listen to someone you care about, and the ability to respond with empathy. All in response to something that is not actually happening to you.

We can see the devolution of memory in these inherited life-or-death memories, which continue to accumulate unchecked. At some point, surely these memories stop being helpful to future generations.

Let me explain a bit more about how this is actually happening.

One client came to see me because he was a bit of a hypochondriac. He was either sick or afraid of getting sick all the time. If anything was going around, he got it. Now, he had never had a major health problem; he tended to catch minor colds and viruses. But he was always convinced that the next illness would be really big. Meanwhile, he had lost jobs because he was out sick so often, and he told me he felt this issue was ruining his life.

What was going on? Did he just have a weakened immune system? Did he get sick because he believed he was going to get sick? Probably yes to both. The real question was, why?

As I do with all my clients, I encouraged him to look into his family history. He talked to several of his relatives, and he discovered that one of his great-great-grandparents, back in the 1800s, lived out on the prairie when he was a little boy with his mom and dad, where there was no doctor within a hundred miles. One day the little boy gets sick. He's not worried about it. He's gotten sick many times before and was always fine after a few days. That's what happens this time, too—he gets better, and everything's fine.

Then, a few months later, Daddy gets sick. Except it turns out Daddy has smallpox and doesn't get better. He dies.

Now, all of a sudden, that little boy's primary belief about getting sick has changed from "no big deal" to "If I get sick, I'm going to die like Dad did." In other words, it becomes a massive life-or-death memory, which the unconscious automatically prioritizes and protects.

The next time that little boy gets sick, he's asking, "Mom, am I going to die like Daddy did?" It makes sense, doesn't it? Even if it makes sense for that little boy at that time, his belief of "If I get sick, I'm going to die" is wrong. And even worse, the new belief that he will die when he gets sick is fear-based, so it activates the stress mechanism in his body, making it far more likely that he will get sick.

As he gets older and gets sick a few more times without dying, his belief might change a little bit, but it will always be there unless the source memory (and its meaning) is completely healed. Until the work to actively reprogram that memory is done, his unconscious mind simply takes control and bypasses his conscious mind. Even though he's got good and bad memories of illness—both recovering from sickness and dying from it—the unconscious mind doesn't care if it overreacts. If it overreacts, he's still alive, which is its number one goal, so it overreacts intentionally. Overreacting is like overachieving for our life-or-death response—it's a good thing! If it underreacts, he may well be dead, violating its prime directive.

Now the fear from this life-or-death memory is infecting every similar memory for the rest of his life. The current situation is coded as a life-or-death memory, and this fear marker keeps spreading like a virus—not just through the boy's own experiences, but passed down to the next generation as well, based on his actions and reactions to illness around him. Because "getting sick" was wrongly programmed with the meaning "I'm going to die" as part of that boy's memory, that memory got protected, prioritized, and passed down. Each generation that received the memory expressed fear, stress, and anxiety when confronted with illness, regardless of how manageable the illness actually was. Each new generation learned to be fearful of illness by watching their mother or father's verbal or nonverbal reactions.

Now, five generations later, my client was born into the world with the same default programming: a deep fear of getting sick, reinforced by observing his own father's extreme effort to avoid getting sick and outsize reaction when somebody else did, which that father observed from his father, and so on. Whenever my client or his family member even sneezes, he's worried the worst-case scenario is going to happen, so he becomes obsessive-compulsive about washing his hands and avoiding germs, or has some other symptom related to the fear of getting sick.

Is that behavior helpful to him now? No! First of all, the original event was that boy's father dying of small-pox, which has been mostly eradicated today. Second, he lives five minutes from the doctor's office, with health insurance and full access to modern medicine. Nevertheless, whenever he feels like he's getting sick, it triggers that danger memory from nearly two hundred years ago, sending fear signals to every cell in his body, causing them to close. The fight-or-flight part of his brain takes control, putting him in survival mode and making him unable to enjoy the present moment, think clearly and creatively, or prioritize what he knows is most important.

Yet because he has no idea where this fear came from, and he has an inherent need to have a reason, he invents a scenario where the fear is a rational response to his cir-cumstances! He cites all sorts of studies about how doing this or that will protect you from the other, and all sorts of news stories about how someone died from a seemingly minor illness. He seeks out information that reinforces what he believes, rather than letting his beliefs be shaped and informed by the reality around him. This is how our unconscious tricks us into believing our inherited beliefs are justifiable and based on evidence. That memory is filtering everything he experiences through an error!

So what did my client need to do to begin to reprogram his memories? First, we worked on healing that inherited memory, which was the source of his issue (and which you'll learn to do in part 2). Once that source memory was healed, we could work on his present-day interpretation of the experience of getting sick. To do that, I began by asking him, "When you think about getting sick now, how do you feel?"

At first, he said, "I feel hopeless. I feel helpless. I feel like the next one is going to be the one that kills me."

But as we continued to work on changing his interpretation of getting sick from a life-or-death situation to something closer to the truth, the less fearful he became.

Eventually, he came in to see me and said, "It has one-eightied."

"What are you talking about?" I said.

"Until I thought about coming here today, I haven't thought or worried about health in two weeks—and I can't ever remember going a day without thinking about health. All of a sudden, it's not an issue for me anymore."

"Well, do you feel sick?" I asked him. He had always felt bad in some way or another when he came to see me.

He paused for a minute. "You know what?" he said.

"I feel great!" He couldn't remember the last time he had felt that way, either.

I checked back in with him six months later, and he had not relapsed at all.

"You know," he said, "it's like that arcade game where you use a big claw to get a prize. Except it's like someone used that claw and just plucked that issue entirely out of my life. It's just gone now."

Your Inherited Memories

Not everybody is going to uncover a devastating ancestral experience that directly traces to an overt fear that you're exhibiting today. Sometimes the history is lost to time; sometimes the precipitating incident isn't literal enough to be passed down. But as you think about your own experiences, consider what experiences your parents, grandparents, or great-grandparents have had in their lives (that you know about). How did they live their lives as a result? Do you see similar reactions in yourself, even though you didn't experience it? If so, it might be a result of inherited memories: through genetics, nurture, or both.

Remember these inherited memories; they'll be helpful to you as you work on re-engineering your own source memories in part 2. And if you have no idea what memory is related to your current situation, we've got you covered there as well.

THE DEVOLUTION OF OUR MEMORIES' MEANINGS

The final area of the devolution of memory is in our interpretations of our memories. With all the life-or-death memories accumulating within our heart over the generations and the availability bias causing us to prioritize negative memories as we experience the world around us, we tend to apply the most negative meaning, or interpretation, to a memory.

Popsicle Memories

A client came to me who was a chronic underachiever. He had graduated at the top of his class in high school, had graduated *summa cum laude* from a top-tier university, and had been recruited by a large marketing firm right after college. He had a clear gift and passion for marketing, but despite all his promise and potential, he could not seem to advance in his job. Whenever he viewed anything as a significant achievement, or something he felt he "had to" succeed at, he would freeze up, not complete the task, and sabotage his own chance at success. This problem showed up not just at work, but in his relationships, too.

As I do with all my clients, I asked him about both his family history and what he remembered most about his childhood. He told me about a time when he was about four years old, where he and his dad were playing soccer in their backyard. It had been a perfect afternoon: lots of goals scored, goals blocked, laughing, and fun. Playing soccer with his dad was one of his favorite things to do.

The sun was beginning to set, and they heard his mom call out, "Come inside for dinner!"

His dad said, "Okay, one more shot for the World Cup!"

My client, the little boy, was overcome with excitement. He kicked the ball as hard as he could—but because he was so excited, the kick went wildly off target, so that his dad had no way to let him win, which he probably intended to.

Laughing, his dad picked him up, and as he was carrying him inside, he said lightly, "You are never going to score any goals if you kick like that! We'll work on it tomorrow."

What would you say if I told you that moment ruined not only that little boy's ability to play soccer for the rest of his life but also his ability to perform in any high-stakes situation?

You probably wouldn't believe me. What in the world did that father do wrong?

Absolutely nothing. Yet my client experienced that event as a trauma just the same, and unless it's healed, it will continue to sabotage positive results in his life.

At age five, the little boy doesn't have the ability to think logically through that statement. Because of our natural negativity and availability biases, and because he's in the delta-theta brainwave state, what instantly gets programmed into his heart is the memory of playing soccer with his dad, missing the shot, and his dad laughing at him and saying he would never be able to score any goals. In other words, he would fail.

He told me that his interpretation of that memory was, "I'm never going to be a good soccer player." To my client at that time, it was the worst thing he could possibly imagine, and he felt like his life was ruined.

I call these kinds of memories *Popsicle memories,* named for one of my clients who was also tremendously intelligent and gifted, and who also couldn't seem to perform well at work. We discovered it all came down to a memory she had from when she was little: her mother gave her sister a Popsicle and didn't give her one. Her mother even said, "Your sister has finished her lunch. When you finish your lunch, you can have a Popsicle, too."

But as a little girl, her interpretation of that event went something like this: "My mom gave my sister a Popsicle and not me because she loves her more. If my mom doesn't love me, that means there's something wrong with me. So when I'm with other people, they're going to know there's something wrong with me, and they're not going to love me either."

Once we healed that memory, she very quickly began to succeed at her job.

I'd be willing to bet any other counselor or psychiatrist would *never* have believed that Popsicle memory was the source of her struggle at work. They'd start looking for repressed memories or hidden "obvious" textbook traumas. But that's exactly what it was. The memory that is shaping your identity may not be an acute trauma. It may be an experience that your memory assigned an enormous amount of power to for reasons you may never fully understand. These Popsicle memories can change the course of your life until you, like my client, can root them out.

What happened next with that little boy? That memory with his dad became the lens through which he experienced every soccer practice and every soccer game. After that, every similar experience triggered a flood of cortisol and adrenaline—not just playing soccer, but any high-pressure situation, anyone laughing at him, any sport he played. The belief "I'm never going to be a good soccer player" dominated his perspective. This experience didn't mean he wouldn't become a good soccer player, but it just got a lot harder. As he got older, this belief was applied to any area of performance. Even though he was gifted in his career area, it became very difficult to succeed there, too.

Many high-performing people, including athletes, believe that stress makes them sharper, and there's nothing wrong with a little stress before a performance. That may be true—for a short time. The release of cortisol and adrenaline from the life-or-death response does flood your muscles with short-term fuel, but after about ten minutes, you start to go into cortisol crash, which makes you more tired than before.

Stress constricts muscles; a stressed muscle becomes tight, and a tight muscle doesn't perform well. That's why you see swimmers and runners at the Olympics "shaking out" their muscles before a race. In tennis, we used to call it "iron elbow"—when the match gets close, you shift to feeling afraid of losing rather than passionate about winning, your elbow gets tight, you can't swing normally, and the ball goes either into the net or five feet out of bounds.

In almost every single Super Bowl game I've seen, the commentators have said it will all come down to which team can relax. When a player or team makes a mistake, they often say they're getting too amped up or too tight.

It's a well-known principle in sports: when it's crunch time, some players step up and play much better, while others don't even hit the rim. It's all based on whether they are *afraid to miss* or *excited to make the shot*. It all depends on what label is on that crunch-time source memory.

And as for the so-called positive boost of energy from stress, non-stress positive hormones can give you an even bigger energy boost without the downside.

That's why stress hurts our performance—not just in sports, but in everything: The report you have to write. Your performance in a play. The important conversation. If you're relaxed rather than stressed, you'll deliver your best performance. What determines whether you're relaxed or stressed? The label on your source memory: whether it's fear-based or love-based.

Together we healed that memory for my client, and he was almost immediately able to execute his ideas at work. Two years later, he told me he received a huge promotion and raise at his company. When he healed the source memory, he was free to perform without stress, in accordance with his gifts, and live up to his full potential in his career.

Are You Afraid of Public Speaking?

When I was a little kid, I loved to sing. One of my favorites was a country music star named Roger Miller, who was very popular at the time, had several number-one hit records, and later won a Tony Award for *Big River*, a Broadway musical he wrote. I especially loved singing two of his songs: "King of the Road" and "Kansas City Star."

I received good feedback, so I kept doing it. Then I did it with a cowboy hat on. Then with a vest and cowboy boots on. Evidently, I had all his little vocal inflections down, and people thought it was cute. I ended up singing those songs in front of my class, then in front of a general assembly at the whole school, and then in front of an assembly of all the schools in the area. It just kept going and going. Finally I was going to sing on live television on Saturday morning on *The Bozo Show*, which was the biggest Saturday morning program at that time. I heard people saying things like, "This guy is going to be the next Shirley Temple."

On Saturday morning, I went to the studio, and *The Bozo Show* was being set up in this great big room packed with people. Well, they didn't take me in there; they took me into a room and closed the door, so I couldn't see or hear the show. It was just me, a camera, and the guy operating the camera. As far as I can remember, they didn't give me any instructions. They just told me to stand there until the time came to sing my song, which in this case was "Kansas City Star."

Obviously I'd never done anything like this in my life, so I just stood there. Then a light on the camera turned on, and the cameraman pointed at me without saying a word.

I was confused. I didn't start singing; I didn't do anything.

I didn't know what was going on. Then he pointed at me again, but I still didn't know what he meant. He pointed at me a third time, and I still didn't know what he meant. Finally, the light went off, and they told me, "Thank you very much. You can go home." Now I was really confused, because I hadn't sung a note.

When I got back to school on Monday, you can imagine what happened. Everyone had known I was going to be on *The Bozo Show,* so they were all tuned in to see me sing that song on television. What they saw was me standing there with my mouth open on live television and never singing a note.

For the next year or so, what I heard was, "Hey, Alex, sing us a song. Hey, Alex, you're the next Shirley Temple, right? Give us a dance. Hey, Bozo!"

I never did anything like that ever again, even though I was asked multiple times. *I am not doing that again. No way.* Around that time I quit singing completely.

A few years later, when I was about fourteen years old, I was told that a group I was in was going to do a presentation, and each of us was going to talk about a different topic for about seven minutes. I didn't really think that much about it until the day of the presentation. I certainly wasn't worried about it.

Let me tell you, when I walked up to that podium, I felt like I was having a heart attack. My knees buckled. My mouth was so dry, I don't think I could have said a word if I wanted to, and I sweated completely through my clothes. Not for a second did I connect this experience to *The Bozo Show,* but that's exactly where it came from. I got up on that stage and my autonomic nervous system said, *No way, get the heck out of here, don't you dare to try to do anything like that again.*

I had never felt like that before in my life. I thought, *What is happening to me? I'm going to literally, physically die right here on this stage.*

Now, of course, I speak in public all the time and don't think anything about it, but I would have never been able to do that if I hadn't healed my memory of The Bozo Show.

Studies show that public speaking is the number one fear on planet Earth—even more common than the fear of death, at least according to our conscious mind. That tells me that most people have errors in their programming that tell their heart that public speaking is going to physically kill them. No one would say public speaking would literally kill them, of course, but, boy, a lot of people feel like they're going to die.

We are not supposed to experience that kind of fear unless our life is in mortal danger. Because of the devolution of memory, public speaking has become the number one fear on the planet when it should not be a fear at all. That doesn't mean you should speak in public if it's not your thing, but either way, it shouldn't trigger your life-or-death response!

If you're afraid of public speaking, be sure you work on that issue when you get to part 2. When you find the source memory and heal it, that fear will just fade away. You'll simply step up onstage, say what you want to say, and sit down. You'll think, "I'm glad I had the chance to share something that's important to me. So, what if they don't like it?"

Inherited Trauma Memories about Identity and Security

We've already mentioned the little boy's traumatized interpretation of his father's death from smallpox: we can understand how witnessing the physical death of someone close to you would lead a child to label that memory with a physical life-or-death label. But life-and-death memories can be generated even when the situation is not literally life or death. Let's return to my own example at the beginning of the chapter, where my mom passed on the memory, "losing my house is going to kill me." Losing her house didn't physically kill her. But in addition to our physical safety, there are at least two other types of memories that can get labeled as dangerous: things that threaten our identity—meaning whether we see ourselves as good or bad—and things that threaten our security, meaning whether we feel safe physically and emotionally or not, and our lives are okay or not okay. Losing her house deeply affected my mother's senses of identity and security.

Here's the problem: the Life or Death label instantly turns on the life-or-death response (fight, flight, or freeze). All the chemicals and responses released in our body and mind are designed to get us to fight, run as fast as we can, or freeze. But when it comes to threats against our identity or security, there isn't a worse response we could have! Why? Our identity and security (based on acceptance or rejection) depend on the health of our relationships. And as we discussed in chapter 1, our relationships were made to run on love—not fear. We'll talk more about this in the next chapter as well.

"Whenever you remember a particular event, your brain releases chemicals similar to those released originally," writes Daniel G. Amen in *Change Your Brain, Change Your Life.*

It's just that most of our remembering is happening unconsciously.

I've seen this effect over and over with my clients. For example, one young woman had been experiencing severe health problems (chronic fatigue and fibromyalgia) as well as severe issues with trust in relationships. My client was a perfectionist and slow to trust. If someone disappointed her, that was it—she never trusted them again, no matter what, and it was often over something trivial. It's very difficult to love and not trust or to do your best without ever making a mistake. She hated the way she was, but she couldn't change it. She knew that her mom and grandma were dealing with similar problems, too.

As usual, I asked her about her family history and her most vivid memories from childhood. That prompted her to ask her mother and grandmother more about their family history, and eventually she discovered that during the Civil War, her great-great-great grandmother's home was attacked by the opposing side. They raped her, killed her husband and children in front of her, and burned her home to the ground. I don't care who you are—you would have trust problems after that. The problem was that her great-great-great granddaughter was still experiencing that same fear when it came to forming trusting relationships. In her current circumstance, my client had no reason to fear relationships. She didn't even know this event had happened until she did some digging in her family history. Again, it wasn't the event that was the problem; it was the inherited memory that said, "Because people raped me, killed my husband and children, and burned down my house, trusting others is going to kill me." *And it was ruining her life.*

The good news is that once my client understood the root of her distrust, she was able to heal it, just as you will learn to do. Her health issues then completely resolved over the next few months.

The Problem Is Never the Problem

I had never had a phone call like this in my life. When I picked up the phone, I heard a voice say, "Hi, my name is Rachel and I do not want to be talking to you."

I thought it was kind of cool, because it was so weird. I thought to myself, *Thank you so much for calling to tell me that. It made my day.*

What I actually said was, "Okay, well . . . what can I do for you?"

"I promised my best friend I would talk to you before I ended my life. So this is my last step." That got my attention!

"I'm so sorry," I said. "Can you tell me what is going on?"

"For three years I've been addicted to all kinds of

drugs—heroin, cocaine, meth—and I've been an alcoholic. For three years, I've been separated from my husband. For three years, my kids don't want to have anything to do with me. For three years, I've been having meaningless sex with anybody and everybody." She'd gone from about 120 pounds to about 80 pounds. She'd been in counseling and therapy. She'd tried everything and was at the end of the road.

I'm not the smartest guy in the world, but when everything she was saying had been going on for "three years," I finally caught on.

"What happened three years ago?" I asked.

"I was raped." Horribly, savagely, in her own home.

"I'm so sorry. Can I ask you what you think and feel when you think about that?"

It was like she pulled a list out of her pocket and started reading it. She didn't have to think about it for a second.

"I feel like a piece of meat, not a person. I feel like I'm dirty in a way that I can never wash it off and be clean again. I feel like I'm not safe, even in the middle of the police station. I can be in a crowd and feel totally alone. I feel like my husband or any other man would never look at me as a desirable woman again. I feel like somehow it was my fault."

"Thank you for telling me this. Let me ask you a question: which of those things you just told me are true?"

She paused. "Well, intellectually I know none of them are true. But they are my twenty-four/seven only reality and I cannot get away from them. It's the only thing I feel. I can't drown them or kill them, and I can't take it any longer."

I knew we had to get the negative environment of her heart more positive, and I believed the best way to start was to bypass the conscious mind, so I started telling her about the Healing Codes, some of the energy tools we'll talk about later in the book.

She told me it sounded stupid.

"Do not think about the memory of the rape," I said. "Just use the energy tool and relax. But, if the memory changes, I think you will know it. If that happens, call me. And call me next week regardless."

She made a sarcastic remark and hung up the phone.

A week later, the phone rang.

"Hi, Dr. Loyd. I want to tell you I did this some last week. I knew it wouldn't work. I just called to tell you I'm done."

I begged her to give it more time, although I didn't think she would.

A week later, the phone rang again. "Hi, Dr. Loyd. I've been doing it. I don't know why I've been doing it, but it didn't work. I know I haven't been very nice to you, so I want to say I'm sorry about that."

That really alarmed me. When people get close to suicide, they often want to make some things right.

"I'm done. Thanks for trying."

I begged her to give it more time.

Four days later, the phone rang, and here's what I hear: sobbing. It was her. She couldn't talk. She was trying to. She couldn't speak; she was just gasping for air, weeping.

Finally, she said, "It changed. It changed. It changed." Still crying.

"I think what you're trying to tell me is that your memory of the rape changed," I said.

"I was doing the code, cursing you out while I was doing it." She really said that.

"I was not thinking about the rape. All of a sudden, the memory of the rape was right in my face in three-D surround sound with the volume turned up high. I couldn't look away.

"For the first time, I looked in the eyes of the man who raped me. I thought, what in the world happened to that man to cause him so much pain that he could do something like that?

"I felt forgiveness, compassion, and pity for the man who raped me. I literally felt it all leave me. All the hatred, the anger, rage, I felt it go. I felt free and I felt like me again."

She immediately stopped all drugs and alcohol, with no withdrawal symptoms. She gained back twenty pounds in the next six months, moving closer to a healthier weight. She reconciled with her husband and children and has been happy and healthy ever since.

That was twelve years ago. I saw her about three weeks ago. She was smiling from ear to ear, sitting on her Harley-Davidson motorcycle, out for a ride. It's one of her favorite things to do.

I'm going to say something that may sound shocking or even offensive, but bear with me. Her problem was never the rape. I'm not saying the rape was not *a* problem; of course it was a problem. But *the* problem was all the lies she was believing related to that event. Her memory of the rape was full of lies. Remember, she told me, "I'm a piece of meat, not a person. I'm dirty in a way that soap can never wash clean. It was my fault. I can never be safe again." She knew it was full of lies from the very first call; she told me on that first call that she knew intellectually that none of those things were true. "The problem" was not the rape, it was the fact that the rape had caused her to internalize demoralizing, demeaning, and evil lies about herself: because I was raped, therefore I'm a piece of meat, etc.

She didn't become an addict and suicidal because of the rape, although every psychologist and medical doctor would say that's exactly why. She became an addict and suicidal because the rape had created beliefs about her identity that were sending a major fear-panic-danger signal to her hypothalamus 24-7.

Your heart does not differentiate between past, present, and future. It treats everything as present-tense reality as if it is happening right now. So, to her heart, she was being raped every hour of every day—with her list of "therefore" meanings associated with it. After three years she couldn't take it anymore.

When that memory healed, did it mean that now she had not been raped or that she couldn't remember it anymore? Of course not! She knew she'd been raped. That part of the memory had not changed at all. The only thing that changed in that memory was the interpretation, the false beliefs that were telling her that the rape was her fault. The memory was no longer telling her that she was bad, or dirty, or inhuman, and the fear signal was no lon-ger being sent to the hypothalamus. After three years of suffering, she was finally able to believe that she was a good person who deserved good treatment, even though something horrific had happened to her.

The lies, in her case, were replaced with peace. Forgive-ness and compassion—both for herself and for the man who had attacked her. Actually, in putting herself in his shoes a little bit, saying if I'd gone through the pain he's gone through, maybe I could have done something terrible, too. You know what we call that? It's the highest level of love. We call it empathy, to literally feel the other person's pain.

After the memory healed, I asked her, "Have you ever felt that way about him before?"

She said, "The only thing I'd thought about him in three years is that I'd like to get a shotgun and blow his head off."

I previously mentioned psychological adaptation and how the human body is equipped to bounce back after virtually any kind of hardship. You may be wondering, why doesn't psychological adaptation kick in when our mind is overreacting and giving the wrong meaning to our memories? Why didn't psychological adaptation work for her?

If every memory has a rating on a scale of negative 10 to positive 10, I believe everyone's heart also has a per-sonal threshold where the negative rating can become too much for psychological adaptation to overcome. For example, this client's overall heart ratio was something like a negative 9—that was beyond her threshold, and psychological adaptation couldn't overcome it. The same was true for my wife, Hope, who was depressed for twelve years.

What can you do for those people whose internal environment is so negative they can't seem to do anything to make their lives better? Somehow you have to get that negative ratio to become more positive, so psychological adaptation can kick in.

That's what memory engineering can do.

THE RESULT: THE DEVOLUTION OF OUR DEFAULT PROGRAMMING

So how about you? Are you feeling negative about certain things in your life that may be a result of this devolution of memory? To find out, try the following exercise.

Recognizing the Symptoms of the Devolution of Memory

Make a list of everything that's bringing up negative feelings like stress, fear, anger, shame, guilt, unforgiveness, frustration, irritation, sadness, or panic. If you search your life, mind, and heart, what are you feeling negative about right now?

Now, for each item on your list, ask yourself: why do you feel that way about those things in your life? For example, maybe you wrote down that you feel irritated at your wife. Why does your spouse irritate you? Maybe he or she always fills the garbage can too full and expects you to take it out. Write that down as well.

Done? Okay.

This was kind of a trick exercise. Unless there was abuse or genuine catastrophe in your lifetime, the real reason you're feeling negative about *all* the situations you listed likely has to do with your unconscious and Popsicle memories, and the devolution of memory that we've been talking about.

This is why you feel overwhelmed. This is why you're tired all the time. This is why you feel stressed too much of the time. You're trying to cope with all this stuff you were never designed to cope with. You were only designed to go into fight-or-flight when your life is truly in danger. But there's been a malfunction in your memories, and your internal fire alarm is going off constantly, for reasons you don't know and that aren't accurate.

Remember the water leak analogy from the introduction. After a few days, the water leaking on the floor may not be so bad. You're able to clean up most of the visible water if you work really hard and get some help. But after ten years, the wood is starting to rot, and your family's getting sick from the mold. Finally, the contractor shows up and tells you your home has been completely devalued or condemned from the damage, and you've lost everything.

None of us come into this world as a blank slate. We all inherit some good from our ancestors, but at this point in history, most of us are significantly affected by the bad: our inherited fear-based programming and beliefs, most of which are no longer helping us. Our strongest, most basic programming is lying to us, so that what we think is real isn't real at all.

I certainly don't know all the trauma memories of my ancestors, and I can't point to every single thing that I learned from my parents. Luckily, I discovered I don't have to know in order to change those memories and see my life truthfully and in a state of love. Neither do you.

But before we can get to healing these source memories, we need to continue the story of how this malfunction happened in the first place. Because this devolution of memory is only the beginning. It only includes the *default* programming we're born with. Once we're born, we begin to add our own memories from our life experience and imagination—all read through this default programming that is wrongly telling us almost everything we see is going to kill us!

(Again, if someone asked if you believed your biggest irritation was literally going to kill you, you would almost certainly answer an emphatic "no." But the truth is that you still *feel* like it's going to kill you; only you've probably gotten so used to it that it seems normal.)

What happens when we start seeing life through the lens of these ancestral memories and start creating exaggerated memories of our own? That's what we'll talk about in the next chapter.

CHAPTER FOUR

The Two Laws

Sometime between ages six and twelve, we make one of the most important decisions of our life. Nearly everyone has to make it alone, and almost no one gets any warning, preparation, or advice about it. And we usually only realize it long after the decision's been made, if at all.

Because of the devolution of memory, nearly everyone is unconsciously programmed to make the wrong choice.

I know I did. Here's how it happened.

Those first, intense experiences of fear and love during and after my birth were my first meaningful memories, although of course I can't remember them consciously. They would also be the first dominoes to set off a long chain of life experiences where fear and love fought for dominance in my life. In fact, I believe the purpose of life is to test us, to see whether we will choose love or fear in any given moment, and more important in our overall life. But to be able to choose, you've got to make sure your definitions of what's life-threatening are the truth.

Later I realized that compared to most people, I have a dramatically "turned-up feeler"—for me, the highs were always higher and the lows always lower. For example, when I was little, I was extremely affectionate. One of my nicknames was "the tree hugger." I'm told that there was a waiting list to babysit me in our town, because they said I was so much fun and so loving to sitters. That was the love part. But pleasure and pain were a much bigger deal to me than other kids I knew—for instance, I constantly wanted things like candy and Coke and felt like I would explode if I didn't get something "NOW!" That was the Law of Externals at work.

I could also sense other people's feelings in a way that almost no one else could. As a very young child, I remember once when my parents' friends came over to visit, and I was in the same general area as their conversation. After they left, I went up to my parents and asked, "Did you know that he was very angry, and that she was really afraid of something?" My parents looked at me as if I were an alien. They hadn't noticed that at all, when it seemed so obvious to me.

About two weeks later, my parents found out this couple—who had put on a great act at our house—was actually going through some truly horrendous circumstances; sure enough, he was angry, and she was afraid.

After that happened, my parents came to me and asked me point blank, "How did you know that?" I thought to myself, *How did you not know that?*

This sensitivity has been a blessing and a curse, kind of like the detective Monk, from the TV series, because it wasn't just sensitivity to others' feelings. My imagination and my feelings were turned way up compared to most people's. Music had an incredibly powerful effect on me. I'd hear a song that really moved me and think, *Wow, this is so powerful!* I'd tell my parents or my friends, "You've got to hear this song!" But when I'd play it for them, they'd say, "Oh, okay, that's nice." Then I realized it didn't affect them at all. The same thing happened with movies and TV commercials. Even today when we're watching movies, Hope or my boys will lean over and ask, "Are you crying again?"

I've been that way my whole life. I've been able to feel other people's feelings, and from what I now know from my doctorate in psychology and my years in counseling, my own feelings are exaggerated in a way that's pretty unusual. It has been a blessing and a curse. It's been wonderful to be more in touch with my own and others' feelings, even though sometimes they're kind of overwhelming. In the counseling setting, I don't know if there's a better gift you can have than the ability to feel other people's feelings. I think that's part of the reason I had a six-month waiting list after six months in practice, when just about every psychologist I knew in the area was only about half full and trying to figure out how to get more clients.

My two older brothers were six and fifteen years older than me, so I had my parents' full attention. I was my dad's main hobby—he would come home every night and every weekend to play with me. My mom would cook whatever meals I wanted and do everything else I could ask. I often wonder if I was spoiled to a much greater degree than a normal baby of the family because of the life-or-death way I came into the world.

So up to about age six, as far as I was concerned, my life was wonderful, even idyllic. It wasn't until I got to school that I realized I was different from the other kids—and not necessarily in a good way. One of my earliest memories on the playground was a boy calling out to me, "Hey, Chunky!" and all the other kids laughing. I laughed, too—and then I went home and cried. That's when I learned I was a bit short and chubby—and that being short and chubby was bad, and it really hurt, even though it had not hurt before.

I felt like I had suddenly been shipped off from the love and safety planet to the fear and danger planet, and it was awful.

Also, even though I was something like a prodigy in the area of feelings and relationships, I must have had every learning disability known to humanity. If I could sum it up, it was like I simply lacked the ability to learn or understand things that were predominantly linear and step-by-step, like algebra and chemistry.

At the end of every school year, there was always the question, "Are they going to let Alex go to the next grade?" Sometimes they did, and sometimes they didn't. I remember one meeting in particular when I was having trouble in every subject and was flunking several of them. The elementary school principal called my mom and me into her office and said, "Alex is a sweet boy. We all love him so much. We don't want you to be worried, because he can learn a trade." They had little hope I'd finish high school, much less college.

At one point, my mom demanded that the school test me. Again, they didn't know about a lot of the learning disabilities they do now, but they did give me an IQ test. It turned out I had a very high IQ. In fact, only two kids in the school had higher IQs than mine, and they both made straight A's. One became a famous neurosurgeon and the other one a rocket scientist.

You'd think this would have made me feel better, but it didn't. It made things much worse. Now instead of "Poor, pitiful Alex," it was, "Alex is lazy." That wasn't right, either! I was great with broad strokes and thinking outside of the box in almost any class or area of life. If they asked me an essay question for which I didn't have to know specific details, I'd blow it away every time. But if I needed to follow lots of rules and minute details, like in grammar, algebra, or chemistry, it was like I was trying to read Russian or something! It just didn't compute at all.

I came to learn later that I was dyslexic and had ADD, ADHD, and probably a couple of other D's they'll discover twenty years from now. Put simply, I thought differently.

I finished last in my high school class; in fact, I didn't know I would graduate until the day before graduation. I had already flunked kindergarten and third grade. (I have been told you can't flunk kindergarten, but I did.)

Sometime during elementary school, I began to shift out

of that delta-theta brain state we talked about earlier, where unconscious beliefs are instantly programmed, and my ability to use my conscious mind started to develop. That meant I could also develop my own beliefs based on my own experience (filtered through my already existing memories, of course). Now, at around age ten, as I kept getting teased day after day for being short and chubby, and I felt stupid academically, negative memory after negative memory began to pile up. One of my beliefs became, "I am fat, and if I continue to be fat, people will continue to be mean and cruel to me, which will cause me to have a bad life." This became the lens through which I experienced a lot of my life, and it created more negative memories in turn.

Note here that I did not create this belief out of thin air. My conscious mind pieced it together based on my memories. That's why changing our conscious beliefs alone doesn't work long-term. Our beliefs come from our memories, and those memories will keep providing the raw material for our beliefs until they're changed—which you'll learn to do in part 2.

THE LIFE VOW

Junior high was probably the worst time of my life. As it began, I was still kind of short and fat, and I also had a pepperoni face, covered with acne. It was also when my oldest brother, who was my hero, had a blow-up with our parents over the family business, and I didn't see him again for forty years.

Because of what happened with my oldest brother, my

parents were in the worst financial struggle of their lives. They thought they might lose the house and go bankrupt; there were a lot of tension and arguments about money and what had happened with my older brother. My mom had one of her fibroid tumor scares at the time, too. They had so much weighing on them that they were mostly oblivious to what was going on with me, flunking school and being made fun of on a daily basis.

At that point, I sort of withdrew from my family. My second older brother got married and moved out of the house, which meant that all of a sudden he wasn't there for me, either.

All of this led to me making a vow one day, sometime around the beginning of junior high: *No one is ever going to make fun of my body again.* I was going to do whatever it took to make sure it would never happen. My negative memories of that experience had built up to the point that people making fun of me felt like it was going to kill me. So, as I saw it, I had four options:

1. Stop caring what people think.
2. Fight them.
3. Run and hide.
4. Exercise like crazy so no one ever makes fun of me for being fat again.

Because of my personality, I dismissed numbers one, two, and three pretty quickly, although I admit I thought about fighting them a lot, to the point that I created

enough internal images of fighting to affect me negatively, almost as if I had actually done it.

I chose option number four. I started running six to
twelve miles a day, doing five hundred to a thousand sit-
ups a day, and a hundred to two hundred push-ups a day.
And guess what—it worked! Hooray for me, right? Well, not
exactly. It's true that people never again made fun of me for
being fat. And yes, I started dating cheerleaders and homecoming queens. But it was all for the wrong reasons. The
changes that I had made to my lifestyle were fear based, not
love based. So instead of joy and peace with my new station
in life, I experienced stress, anxiety, and obsession. I *had* to
do this excessive exercise every day no matter what—I really
did feel like I would die if I didn't, even for just one day.

I call these decisions *life vows*. Almost every addictive
cycle I've seen, where someone simply can't use their
conscious choice to stop doing something they don't
want to do or start doing something they want to do, can
be traced back to a life vow.

A life vow is when you reach a point of so much pain
that you swear that you will never be in that particular circumstance again. You will do whatever it takes to
avoid it in the future, no matter how much it costs.

For example, you grow up in a home where your
parents scream at each other, and you vow, *I'll never be in a
house where there is screaming again.* You do everything you can
possibly do to avoid making anyone angry or even mildly
irritated with you, but at least no one is screaming. You
may not experience screaming, but you're also missing

out on great joy, laughter, and relationships with intimate intensity. The cure ends up being worse than the sickness.

Life vows can have even more severe consequences. One of my clients grew up in a little town on what they used to call "the wrong side of the tracks." Her dad left her and her mom when my client was eight, and they were poor by any definition. Her mom also got the reputation of being "easy."

As a young girl, my client made a Scarlett O'Hara–type vow, much like I did: "With God as my witness, I will never be poor again." She became obsessed with money and external things, and she had the worst stress and anxiety I had ever seen. She would never do what I asked her to do to heal, because she couldn't let go of the externals.

She was eventually diagnosed with terminal cancer and died at age thirty-nine. Her doctors said it was likely from all the stress and anxiety, and I knew the source of that stress: it was the life vow she made as a result of her childhood. The real problem had nothing to do with money but with her memories growing up.

Exercise

Can you remember making a vow like mine when you were a child or teenager? Was something so painful that you finally decided you would do whatever it took to make sure it never happened again?

Nearly everyone has had this kind of experience somewhere in their lives. And what we don't realize is that in that moment, our choice is setting up a chain reaction that can cause everything in our lives to malfunction from that point on. The only question is how long it will take for the weakest link to break.

That's exactly what happened to me when I vowed that no one would ever make fun of my appearance again. At the time, it seemed like my only choice if I wanted to have any kind of success in life. It took years before I realized I even had a choice, and I had made the wrong one. By then I had already broken at my weakest link, as you'll see in the next chapter.

THE MOST IMPORTANT CHOICE

What choice am I talking about? I'm talking about the choice between following the Law of Externals or the Law of Internals.

As I said in chapter 1, the Law of Externals says that our external circumstances are the most important thing, beginning with our physical survival and extending to any other circumstance that would cause us pleasure or relieve pain. It is rooted in our survival instinct, and it's the system of "the ends justify the means," of pursuing "what I want when I want it." It's the system of natural law, specifically the law of cause and effect, and it is absolutely real.

The intention is to get the end results that benefit you, even if it means others have to lose or get hurt. It means prioritizing your own needs over others, and self-protection over relationships. It's living a life of seeking pleasure and avoiding pain. The governing motive is *fear*.

As I explained in chapter 1, the Law of Externals has a very important positive purpose: it's meant to unconsciously govern our decision making from birth until our conscious mind develops. It makes sense that we're wired to focus on externals as children, because we are more likely to physically die from accidental death (i.e., from externals) during that time than any other time in our life. Children need to speak up if they're cold, hungry, unwell, or unbalanced. For any parent who has been up with a hungry baby in the middle of the night, you know that baby doesn't care how tired you are—he or she is going to make sure you know that it's time to eat! We need our heart's survival instinct in control of our actions and decisions if we expect to live to adulthood!

But once our prefrontal cortex develops to the point where we are capable of logical thought and conscious choice, we have the capacity for more. Now we're capable of putting aside our personal comfort and self-interest for the greater good when our physical life is *not* in danger—and making win-win-win decisions.

In other words, we are capable of living according to the Law of Internals. The Law of Internals has us evaluate ourselves by our internal state rather than our external circumstances. The Law of Internals guides us toward an internal state of love over the internal state of fear. Our operating principle for the Law of Internals is not our survival instinct but our conscience. When we follow the Law of Internals, we no longer prioritize pursuing personal pleasure or avoiding personal pain, as we did when we lived under the Law of Externals; instead, it leads us to take pleasure in pursuing the highest good for all parties involved. The governing motive is love.

As I explained in chapter 1, as children under the Law of Externals, ideally we have parents or caregivers who are operating by the Law of Internals and bathing us in love, giving us ten instances of positive feedback for every negative. Unfortunately, either consciously or unconsciously, we are exposed to beliefs about the world that lead us to doubt the security of the Law of Internals and to believe that if we do not put our own needs first that we will be left with nothing. Very understandably, we choose the Law of Externals, the law of prioritizing pleasure or avoiding pain in every decision, and the law that says our external circumstances are what matter most.

If we continue to choose to seek pleasure and avoid pain, if we continue to value self-preservation above all else, if we do not overcome fear, we continue to live according to the Law of Externals.

Most parents never have this conversation with their kids about the system that governs their decision making and priorities, even though it's so incredibly important. The reason is obvious: most parents don't know it exists, either. So, when kids have the ability to choose what law to live by, most parents have a talk with their kids that goes something like this: "Well, you're getting older now. It's time to take responsibility for your life, and learn how to get the results you want." And then they teach them whatever they think will help their child get the results they think are most important.

These parents love their kids. They're not trying to ruin their lives. They just don't know about the Law of Internals, which is actually the only way for them to get the best results in their lives.

In fact, we've never needed the Law of Internals more. In the previous chapter, I mentioned a self-help thought leader who teaches that the secret of life is self-interest. He's actually a great friend of mine, even though we teach opposite things. I've probably got thirty or forty friends like that around the world—we teach and believe very different things, but we stay in each other's homes, greet each other with genuine hugs. I have no animosity at all toward them.

Contrast that with the current political climate in the United States since 2016, where people seem to absolutely hate those who disagree with them.

If you choose to live by externals, that's the end result.

If you choose to live by internals, you have friends like mine, where you can freely disagree (and even deeply disagree), but still have close, respectful, loving relationships. You might even learn something.

I have a friend who is influential in the political world, and he tells me, whether Democrat or Republican, politicians tend to huddle in back rooms, lick their finger and see which way the wind of public opinion is blowing, and say whatever that is. Their statements and policy decisions often have little to do with what they believe is good or best.

That's the Law of Externals in action. That's a result of living in fear.

On the other hand, I think of political leaders like Abraham Lincoln, who would sometimes have rotten vegetables thrown at him when he spoke in public. But as best I can tell, he always tried to do what he thought was right, regardless of public opinion.

We've lost that quality in much of our leadership, and we need it desperately—not just for our individual well-being, but for the future of our families, our nations, and our world.

Parenting According to the Law of Internals

If you're in the thick of parenting right now, you may be wondering, *How do I help my children avoid making life vows and choose the Law of Internals rather than the Law of Externals when the time comes? When do you provide consequences—even kind consequences—and when do you just forgive?*

I think you absolutely follow the law of cause and effect as a parent when your kids are younger. But while teaching them about the physical world and ensuring their survival, bathe them in love and 10 positives to one negative. Loving discipline and instruction, not just discipline.

Remember, those first six to twelve years, when our brain is primarily in a delta-theta state, we're supposed to be living under the Law of Externals. Then, after that age, we are able to shift into a beta brain state, where we become capable of learning to live by what is right, regardless of the pain or pleasure result. We become capable of delayed gratification, and even choosing pain over pleasure at times. (The beta brain state is also where we are capable of experiencing stress, and where most adults live most of the time.) That's when our parents can start teaching us the Law of Internals, and how to choose it at home, at school, and on the playground, and how to put it into action more and more.

Teaching the Law of Internals is not a matter of following a list of specific rules, though. I remember when my first son, Harry, was born. I never had any apprehension about being a parent—until I saw him in the nursery. All of a sudden, a wave of extreme fear came over me. I thought, *This little guy is going to be looking to me to make all the right decisions in life. I can't do this! I'm going to screw it up.*

I said a little prayer, and I had a very clear thought that I believed was from God: *Alex, if he knows 100 percent, beyond a shadow of a doubt, that he is loved exactly the way he is, faults and all, then you will have done okay. That's all you have to do.*

I felt all my anxiety melt away. I thought, *Okay. Maybe I can do that.*

That has been my north ever since: making sure my kids know they are loved 100 percent, no matter what they do. I believe that single principle is the secret to parenting, and to making sure your kids will transition to the Law of Internals when they're able.

For example, with my sons, I would ask them repeatedly:

What could you do that would cause me to love you more?

Nothing.

What could you do that would cause me to love you less?

Nothing.

Today I just need to say the first few words and they finish it for me.

If your kids know this one thing, most other things will work themselves out.

And it's okay if you mess up. If you yell at them for breaking something, just sit down with them later and apologize. You can say, "I'm sorry. I was irritated, and that irritation had nothing to do with you. I shouldn't have yelled at you when you broke that glass. I love you no matter what."

I was having a conversation with a renowned psychologist and bestselling author one day, and he said that some parents came to him and were having problems with their kids. "I just don't understand it," they said. "We raised them all exactly the same way."

"Well, that was the problem," he told me. "They raised them all exactly the same way, when no two kids are the same."

Rather than follow a list of parenting rules (with the possible exceptions of not screaming at your kids and not hitting them), instead your guiding principle is, "What can I do in this particular situation that will help my child know they are loved exactly as they are, 100 percent, no matter what they do?" That will be different for every kid, and it may even differ by the day.

When I tell parents this, I often hear, "Wait a minute—what about discipline?" Well, I'm all for discipline! Just discipline in a loving way. Provide natural and loving consequences, which means the consequences aren't given in anger or to hurt the child because their actions hurt you in some way. Watch your tone and body language, which kids can read easily.

If you're a parent of older kids, start teaching them about delayed gratification and doing what's right, even if it hurts temporarily. You can make it a game and give them a choice: "You can have ten minutes to play video games right now, or one hour of video games later, and I'll play with you." If they choose instant gratification, don't get mad—give them a hug. Be loving and kind. Remember that what is valuable enough to cause a child to choose delayed gratification is different for each child. After choosing delayed gratification fifty times or so, they're now programmed to choose it, and you don't need the game anymore.

And if you're a parent of a teenager or young adult and you know they're capable of delayed gratification, you can start shifting into the Law of Internals completely and release them from punishment. Treat them as the adult they are.

I have messed this up more than I've got this right. But I'm still trying.

However, because of the devolution of memory, even if we are taught truth and love, we may not see it. The errors in our memories may be distorting everything so that fear and lies are our default. Because we're raised by parents and a society living according to the Law of Externals, many of us don't even know there's any alternative. As a result, many of us don't even know the difference between love and fear. We may say the word "love" all the time, as I did, but only understand love as positive feelings for others as long as I'm getting what I want and they aren't interfering with that. Or we just say the word because others do, and we feel it helps us get what we want. If that's true, we will always feel that something is missing, like we aren't good enough, like we can't be safe just being who we are, because we aren't experiencing real love. We're just experiencing "what's in it for me" love.

So when we hit adolescence and the time comes to choose which system we're going to live by, the vast majority of people (in my experience) continue on the path to seek pleasure/avoid pain and end up in the Law of Externals—a system based on the lie that you're constantly in crisis—which governs your thinking to believe that you're in danger, that you need to always prioritize what's in it for you, and that leads you in the opposite direction of greater meaning and higher purpose. In essence, your conscious mind has been tricked by the illusion of constant danger signals from your unconscious, and you don't even realize it.

That's what happened to me when I made my life vow to never get ridiculed for my body again. I was going to do whatever it took to change my external circumstances so I would never experience that kind of pain again. I chose to live by the Law of Externals.

I believed the external was causing me pain, but it was actually my internal state. I had made a wrong interpretation of my external circumstances: I believed that if I was fat, or had pimples, or was ugly, I was a horrible person and could not be loved. That is never the case. Our externals never determine our internal value.

If you try to get internal worth through external circumstances, you'll likely never get it.

On the other hand, if you focus on listening to your conscience, which inherently knows that you are valuable regardless of external circumstances, you almost always get the internal state of love and self-worth *and* the externals you want.

If you've been operating primarily by the Law of Externals for your entire life, that might sound like nonsense. How can we get the external circumstances we want if we don't focus on them? How can we not prioritize external goals like finding a place to live, a life partner, a job? To do otherwise seems like a path straight to losing everything that matters.

If we choose the Law of Externals instead of the Law of Internals as adolescents (which is when it usually happens), it means we believe external circumstances will give us the internal state of love, joy, and peace that we want. In other words, we expect external results to "buy" us happiness. When we graduate from school, then we'll be happy. When we find a partner who truly loves us, then we'll be happy. When we buy that big-screen TV, a bigger house, that tropical vacation, then we'll be happy. When we finally earn that platinum album or get on the New York Times bestseller list, then we'll be happy.

But will we?

Clint Gresham played for the Seattle Seahawks when they won the Super Bowl in 2013. According to Gresham, it was a day he would never forget. But as the days and weeks passed, he said that he and his teammates were waiting for it to sink in that they won the Super Bowl. In other words, they were waiting for winning the Super

Bowl to give them the permanent happiness they had expected it to. It never happened.

"Was it awesome winning a Super Bowl? Absolutely. Did it make me happy and satisfy my core need for significance, joy, love, or value? Not even close," concluded Gresham.

Gresham and the Seahawks returned to the Super Bowl in 2014—and lost. According to Gresham, losing was incredibly painful, but as he puts it, "The idea of running from our pain is actually what is destroying our world. It's only in your pain that you can grow."[1]

My friend William Tiller, PhD, renowned Stanford University physicist, tells me that in physics, the unseen is always the parent of the seen, and never the other way around. The same is true for our lives. No visible, external circumstance can give you internal happiness long term. Only the internal state of love can do that. The internal is always the parent of the external, and never the other way around.

EXPECTATIONS ARE A HAPPINESS KILLER

Let's take a deeper look at what's happening when we choose the Law of Externals, and specifically at expectations.

Your prefrontal cortex has a function called your *experience simulator*. It allows you to imagine doing something, picture how it is likely to turn out, and then decide to do it, or not. To "try it before you buy it," so to speak. That picture becomes your *expectation* of what will happen.

You may not be at all conscious of creating that future

expectation. We do it so naturally that it happens without us realizing it, or it's done unconsciously. Before you do anything at all, even brush your teeth, your mind creates a picture of what it expects to happen before you do it.

However, the latest research tells us that our experience simulator lies to us a lot of the time. For example, the research of Harvard professor Daniel Gilbert, PhD, has shown that humans are terrible at accurately predicting how they will feel and what will happen concerning something in the future.

In one study at Harvard University, he and his team asked student participants about their expectations in certain imaginary scenarios. For example, if you bought a piece of art today, would you be buying it for your pleasure now or because it may be worth double in ten years? If you were going on a date, would you be thinking about having a good time in the moment or what would happen after the date?

They found not only that the participants were likely to have expectations about what would happen in the future, but also that those expectations killed their happiness in the *present*. Why? Expectations focus on the future, not the present, and you can only experience happiness in the present.

That's why Gilbert calls expectations a "happiness killer."[2] If you read the full scope of his research, expectations kill much more than happiness. They kill your health, success, relationships, and virtually everything else, because expectations cause your body to be flooded with life-or-death stress chemicals every time something doesn't go the way you expect.

How? If you follow the Law of Externals and believe your internal self-worth, identity, security, or happiness depends on a specific external result, you create an expectation of that result. The instant your reality doesn't match that expectation, your hypothalamus pulls the stress fire alarm. And the whole process is typically doomed from the start, because the original assumptions are erroneous. So the end result is that whatever you do to try to make your life better actually makes it worse—over and over again.

Let me illustrate with an everyday example. Imagine you've decided to go to the grocery store to get your favorite brand of frozen pizza for dinner. You can already taste it! The grocery store is only about five minutes away.

You head out to your car—but your car won't start. How would you feel? Calm, cool, and collected—or frustrated?

Most people would experience something in the anger family, anywhere from irritated to downright livid. That's a sign your heart has decided this is a matter of life and death, pulled the fire alarm, and sent out the Fear Response Team.

Let's say you get the car started and on the way you hit traffic. Your heart pulls the fire alarm again.

Then a massive downpour hits. *Oh, crap,* you think. Fire alarm!

You park your car, and while walking through the parking lot to the store, you step in a pothole full of water. Fire alarm!

When you get to the frozen section, you discover they're out of your favorite brand of pizza. Fire alarm!

You have just one item, but only two checkout counters out of twelve are open, and there are twelve people in each line. Fire alarm!

You hit traffic again on your way home. Fire alarm!

Finally, you get home and cook the pizza. It doesn't even taste good! Fire alarm again.

That experience might have ruined your whole evening, if you were like I used to be. Or if you're like my wife, Hope, used to be, it might take you three days to recover!

Your negative reactions to all these external circumstances meant that your experience simulator was picturing and expecting the opposite. When you imagined "going to the grocery store to buy a frozen pizza," your experience simulator was picturing the car starting, no rain, no potholes, the store having an ample supply of your favorite brand of pizza, fast checkout, an easy drive home, and a perfectly cooked pizza.

Negative reactions come when expectations do not align with reality. And when the experience simulator is too rigid and doesn't leave room for variation, it triggers the fear response system for things that are simply just a different way of getting to the end goal. The problem isn't that there was rain and traffic and crowds and a change to the dinner menu; the problem is that your experience simulator responded to minor changes in the programming by completely breaking down.

This is what your experience simulator is doing not

just for your trip to the grocery store, but for your job, your kids' behavior, your significant relationship, and pretty much everything else that's part of your life.

And if you believe your internal state of love, joy, and peace depends on getting those specific external circumstances, then if you don't get them, you'll never be happy. In fact, you won't be happy long term even if you do get the desired result, because that happiness won't last.

Under the Law of Externals, we create these kinds of experiences for ourselves all the time. And then we wonder, *Why am I never at peace?*

But in addition to taking away your internal peace, the Law of Externals can take away the external results you want as well.

When I was in my twenties, I had just been hired at a new job, and my supervisor was super driven and super perfectionist. I kept this to myself, but it was clear to me that she was compensating for low self-worth by acting as if she had very high self-worth. In fact, it seemed very important to her that everyone know she was better than everyone else, as she constantly talked about her achievements, large or small.

It turned out she didn't like me because she couldn't control me. My job was to work with teenagers and their parents, and she wanted me to wear a suit and tie and sit in the office from eight to five on weekdays. I knew I wouldn't be able to do my job effectively that way, so I wouldn't do it. I told her boss about what was going on, and he told me I didn't have to do what she was demanding. From then on, she wanted me gone. Eventually she started telling lies about me to my boss, which ultimately got me fired.

After I left, the truth came out, and she got fired—not only fired, but humiliated, because it came out that she had been telling lies about many other things for years.

The Law of Externals is not a sustainable way of living. Eventually, it will lead to trouble—either by failing to get you any more of what you want or by jeopardizing all that material stuff that you were using it to accumulate in the first place.

THE LAW OF INTERNALS GETS YOU THE INTERNALS AND THE EXTERNALS YOU WANT

In contrast, following the Law of Internals is the only way to be satisfied internally *and* externally.

I had one client who flew in to see me from Los Angeles based on a referral. He was a celebrity in the music industry, a multi-multimillionaire, a type A personality, and the most unhealthy person I had ever known. His lifestyle included regular drugs and alcohol and cheating on his wife, and he was constantly paranoid about losing the steady flow of millions of dollars coming from shady financial deals.

His doctor had just told him he would probably be dead in ten years from a chronic disease. He was stunned. He had believed his life was the absolute road map for happiness.

He didn't see anything wrong with his behaviors. "Have you ever tried cocaine?" he asked me. "What a rush!" Why wouldn't he have relations with beautiful young women, even when he's married? "Anyone would if they could," he bragged. He owned multiple boats, ropes of gold jewelry, and a $250,000 Ferrari.

I discovered that his pursuit of this lifestyle was intentional: he had grown up in a poor neighborhood, his family often didn't have enough money, and he decided that no matter what, he was going to have it all. He was flabbergasted that he was unhappy and unhealthy, because from his perspective, he truly did have it all, which was why he had come to see me.

Now it was my turn to be flabbergasted. The first thing I said was, "There's a 99 percent chance that when I tell you this, you're going to run out of my office like your hair's on fire."

Then I told him about the Law of Internals and Externals, the importance of prioritizing relationships above results, memory engineering in the form it existed at that point, and energy work.

He never actually ran out, but his body language told me he wanted to. Instead, he paid me, thanked me, and left.

I thought I'd never see him again. Six months later, he came back.

"I have been trying everything in the world to avoid needing to come back and do what you suggested," he said. "It goes against everything I vowed. But I think maybe you are right."

We worked on reengineering his memories and practicing the Law of Internals rather than the Law of Externals. It was very difficult for him, but he stuck with it.

A year later, when he came to see me for his last visit, he was still rich and still famous. But other than that, he was a different person. His hair and clothes were less flashy. He was off drugs and cut way back on alcohol. He started treating the people who worked for him more kindly and started paying them more. Rather than easily getting angry at those closest to him, he became kind. He was night and day happier and healthier.

At the end of our session, he thanked me. "Never in a million years did I think I'd be happier this way," he said. "But I am."

But the ones who were the most thankful were his wife, housekeepers, yard keepers, and accountants. They saw the difference most clearly and benefited greatly as well.

That's an extreme example. My specialty was relationships, so I also saw a lot of couples who were close to divorce. I used to say if I could get one of them, I'd get both of them. Even when only one person changes, the entire relationship can change for the better very quickly, much like touching one part of a baby mobile changes the location of every other part.

I had a client recently who was married to the same woman for thirty years. Their marriage was great for the first six months, then it was okay for about twenty years, and then in the last ten years they had been more like roommates. My client also told me that he would never tell his spouse this, but if he could do it all over again, he would never have chosen to be in a committed relationship with her.

I learned that his dad died relatively young at age

forty-five, and his mom never really recovered. He was the oldest and therefore became a parent to his siblings. His mother developed a bad reputation in town, and many kids at school made fun of him because of his mom. His life vow became, *I'm going to have a respectable family.*

As a result, after he was married, he became very controlling with his wife: what she wore, whom she interacted with, where she went each day. He truly believed she was sneaking around, cheating on him or lying to him. No matter how many times she denied it, he didn't believe her, and he would sometimes secretly follow her. What came across to her was that he didn't trust her. Her interpretation was, *If he doesn't trust me, he must not love me, even though he says he does.*

I explained the difference between the Law of Externals and the Law of Internals, and I gave him the tools to work on his fear-based memories so he was capable of choosing the Law of Internals. Once he healed his fear-based memories that kept him stuck in the Law of Externals, he did choose to live by the Law of Internals, and he started applying it to his biggest issue: his marriage. For the first time, he made the connection between what he experienced with his father and mother and how he was acting in his marriage.

He had honestly been worried his wife was cheating on him, but when he reengineered the fear-based memories that were distorting his perspective, he saw the situation very differently. Most important, he was able to empathize with her. If you're in a lot of internal pain, it's very hard to empathize.

Once he saw the situation from her perspective, his focus shifted from trying to control externals to benefit himself to simply showing love to his wife. Before, he never did much to show love except to tell her he loved her and work at his job to help support the household. Now, he would reach down to hold her hand or touch her arm gently during the day. What made the biggest difference to his wife—she started crying when she told me this—was his tone of voice.

"When he talks to me now, he has a tone of voice I haven't heard since we were dating," she said. "His tone is kind, and it tells me that he is interested in my opinions."

We know that most communication is nonverbal. For example, FBI detectives are trained in reading microexpressions, and I'm told you can't fake them. Before, his body language, tone, and microexpressions were saying, "I love me—do this for me." Now, according to his wife, they were saying, "I love you, and I value you." Period. He wasn't trying to change his nonverbals, of course— they were evidence of the internal change.

They held a recommitment ceremony, and he apologized for all those years of suspecting her, telling her, "It was never you. It was me." Their trust was rebuilt.

Now he is telling everybody he knows that there's another way to live, and living according to the Law of Internals is the most important thing in his life. He told me, "You know, when I really think about it, it's not rocket science. Instead of doing things so that we'd avoid arguing or so she would treat me a certain way, I do things for her a hundred percent just because I love her. What I do has nothing to do with equilibrium or how she will treat or think about me. We've got a relationship now that's even better than our first six months of marriage, and I never asked her to change a thing. But what I changed changed everything."

It's a common psychological axiom that we tend to see in others the negative issues we have within ourselves. What you hate in someone else might just be a reflection of the toxicity of your own heart. When your internal toxicity is healed, the way you see the situation changes. What used to be an absolute deal-breaker becomes something you want. If your heart is too toxic, you could find something to hate about Mother Teresa. Be careful about judging others and acting on it until you know your own heart is healed.

Another client, a thirty-five-year-old woman, also had an issue with trust. She had recently divorced her husband, which had absolutely devastated her. She seemed to be one of those sweet, innocent, kind people about whom you'd wonder how anyone could leave her.

When I asked more about how she grew up, I learned that she was raised to believe that there were only two kinds of people: good or bad, and you had to be good or you'd go to hell and your life would fall apart. A long list of regulations determined whether she was a good girl or a bad girl, which had to do with the way she dressed, religious beliefs, how much makeup she could wear, what she could do with boys, etc.

She met and married a man, and her biggest priority

was pleasing her husband and being a good mom—so she could be a good girl. Even though she was doing a lot for others, it was really all about her—doing certain external actions for her self-worth and identity. Eventually she got frustrated: not surprisingly, she couldn't do everything right, but if she did something wrong or her husband got irritated with her, she felt like a bad girl.

A few years into the marriage, her husband had an affair, and it devastated her. She was experiencing anxiety and depression and wanted nothing to do with other men. After what happened to her, she felt she could never trust another man again.

I explained the Laws of Internals and Externals to her. The science and theory made sense to her, but I vividly remember that she started crying when I told her about choosing the Law of Internals. I asked her, "Don't you want love in your life again?"

"Yes, I want that more than anything," she said, "but I can't trust anyone!"

"Why can't you trust anyone?"

"Because they might hurt me."

In other words, she couldn't control them.

The hardest thing about living according to the Law of Internals was giving up control. It was like I had asked her to take a pair of pliers and pull her own teeth out.

It was a long and difficult process. We had to do a lot of memory engineering and energy work to heal all the negativity that had built up in her heart since childhood and the feeling that she needed to control every aspect of her life in order to have any sense of self-worth. We uncovered a lot of rage and anger as well.

Then, after about three months, she became capable of letting go of control and choosing the Law of Internals. That began three more months of going back and forth between the Law of Externals and the Law of Internals, of trying and stumbling and trying again.

Finally, after about six to eight months, her memories were healed, and she had fully made the shift. She became the sweet, kind lady I knew she was when she first came in, inside and out.

I saw her a few months ago, which was a few years after we had worked together. She was now in a relationship with a nice, loving guy, and she was just beaming.

She gave me a hug, and here's what she told me: "This is the only thing I've ever found that is a guaranteed miracle for everything I apply it to. Even my external circumstances start blooming in a way they never bloomed before, no matter how hard I tried to make them bloom. The only difference is that now they bloom without me trying to do anything."

That's the typical result of the Law of Internals.

I hope you notice that the key in all of these situations was not about changing their external circumstances. I'm not saying external circumstances don't need to be changed or that you shouldn't change your external circumstances. If clients were in abusive situations, I told them to get the heck out of there, and most of the time they did. I'm simply saying that most people put the cart

before the horse: if you try to change your external circumstances first, you might be working against yourself,
because you probably won't be able to do it.

If I could sum up what the Law of Internals looks like
in action, it would be *empathy*. By empathy, I don't mean
feeling someone else's pain because their pain affects
you. I mean being able to put yourself in another person's
shoes whose experience has nothing to do with you.
Rather than following the Golden Rule—treat others the
way you want to be treated—you are able to follow the
Platinum Rule: treat others how *they* want to be treated.

Exercise

What law are you living under: the Law of Externals or the Law of Internals?

I've found that many people have a hard time
knowing which system they're living in, because
most people who live under the Law of Externals
have also tried their best to incorporate love into
that system.

Remember the results of the Law of Externals.
If you keep trying to choose love while under this
law, you'll end up in constant stress and eventually
break at your weakest link.

Also, two people living according to different
laws can look and act exactly the same... until
something doesn't go their way.

Here's one way to know what law you're living by: are you able to put yourself in another person's shoes and treat them the way they want to be treated, even when it doesn't directly benefit you or may inconvenience you? In other words, are you able to empathize with someone even if what happens to them doesn't affect you at all?

If not, you're likely living according to the Law of Externals.

If you are living according to this law, do you remember choosing it?

It could have happened in a couple of ways: maybe there was a time in your life when out of pain, boredom, or a desire for pleasure, you violated your own belief system, and it turned into a cycle of repeatedly doing that forbidden thing to avoid pain or get some kind of pleasure.

Or maybe you did what I did, and made a *Gone with the Wind* kind of vow: "With God as my witness, I'll never be hungry again." "I'll never be fat again." "I'll never be hurt by someone else again."

Or rather than choosing it, did you simply keep using the software program you were born with, saw modeled by those close to you, and were more or less comfortable in?

Let's finish our explanation of the Great Memory Malfunction. If you've chosen the Law of Externals, like most people have and I certainly did, the malfunction doesn't end there. Living under this law effectively puts you in a state similar to some degree of physiological shock, with your best decision-making abilities inaccessible to you. No wonder it's so hard to do what you know is best! And that's the topic of the next chapter.

CHAPTER FIVE

Why You Can't Do What's Best for You

After I made that vow that no one would ever make fun of my appearance again, chose to seek pleasure and avoid pain, and committed to the Law of Externals, I did exactly what I said I was going to do. And it was horrible.

As I mentioned in the previous chapter, over the next twenty years of my life, I worked my way up to running six to twelve miles and doing 300 push-ups and at least 500 sit-ups every single day, no matter what. I watched what I ate. I did what I could to clear up the acne.

Before that, the pretty girls didn't pay me any mind at all. After that, I was dating cheerleaders and homecoming queens. But it was totally for the wrong reason.

My focus on weight and fitness became a massive addiction, an obsession, really. Every day I would go into the bathroom, pull my shirt up, and look in the mirror: *Do I have any fat anywhere, is there anything sticking out over my belt even a little?* I would evaluate those things probably six to eight times a day. I believe I was almost anorexic.

If I had a super-busy day and it looked like I wasn't

going to get to run that night, man, I would almost be in a panic. *I'm going to be fat. I'm going to be fat. I'm going to be fat!* Well, of course I wasn't going to be fat after missing one day, especially not when I ran thirty miles over the last four days and was watching what I ate!

The next day, I would usually starve myself trying to make up for it, and maybe run fifteen miles instead of six to twelve. Yet I still felt like that wasn't enough, which makes no rational sense at all, because it was more than enough. But if I missed even one day, it would probably take me ten days until I felt like I had made up for it.

I knew I was addicted. I hated it, but I couldn't stop it. I was addicted to the payoff.

I was also caught in a cycle of inferiority and superiority, which always comes from the Law of Externals. On one hand, I was terrified of being fat again. It truly felt like it was a matter of life or death, and it had me in a constant state of anxiety, addiction, or inferiority. On the other, if I was doing well, I had this feeling of superiority. But understand, my definition of "fat" was totally ridiculous—one ounce more than I weighed yesterday.

I was always either low or high. I was never at peace.

I know people today who would look at that situation as a success. I achieved my goal. But every person I know who would interpret it this way is miserable themself in some area of their life, and evaluates their own lives by the externals.

Of course, I'm not saying that exercising and watching what you eat is a bad thing. When I realized I wanted to change the way I looked, I could have said, "You know what? I'm going to get in shape. And because it's good for me, I think I'll be happier. Maybe people will quit making fun of me, but that's not the main reason I'm doing it. And if I miss a day, I miss a day. No big deal." I could have done very similar things while prioritizing an internal state of love, I would probably have had even better external results, and I would have been at peace.

But I didn't. I wasn't able to. Hope would tell you in two seconds, "It was an obsession. It was not healthy. It was way over the line. There was no joy in it." Sure, I enjoyed dating pretty, nice girls, but there was always this underlying anxiety and addiction keeping me from enjoying it the way I could have.

Later, I had to have double hip replacements. Guess why? I beat my body to death, almost literally, because of this extreme terror of being mocked, of people calling me names and girls wanting nothing to do with me, and of how much that hurt.

Pay attention to why you're wishing for what you're wishing for and how the idea of getting it makes you feel. I got exactly what I wished for, I just didn't expect what would come with that. I thought I was making the best decisions I could. What I didn't know was that I was actually living in an illusion, a fear-based simulation created by erroneous memories, and my survival response was controlling everything I thought, believed, felt, and did. I had no access to the parts of me that actually knew what was best, because in my pain I refused to listen.

Yet that was only the beginning. By the time I was in my twenties, every area of my life began to fall apart, including my health—and I couldn't seem to do anything about it.

Hope and I met in college, started dating just after college, and got married about a year or so later. Being married has been the hardest thing I have ever done in my life. One of the wisest premarital counselors I've ever known said that he tells everyone he counsels this about marriage: God picks the one perfect person in the world to kill you dead.

He said, "Every single time I say that, they chuckle. 'Haha, that's a good one!' I say, 'I'm not joking. That is not a joke.' Then they say something like, 'Okay, yeah, yeah, yeah, we know. Marriage is really hard. Everybody says it's really hard.'"

Then they leave, and he thinks to himself, *They don't have the first clue.*

He said it's so predictable. Usually about six months later, the wife calls him or comes to see him and says, "How did you know?" Now, six months later, she feels like she's being killed dead. So does he.

The brilliant therapist that I did one of my doctoral internships under, Dr. Gale Napier, said that when two people get married they each push their invisible shopping cart of junk down the aisle. Nobody sees it or smells it or anything. It's completely invisible. Then, after about six months, it starts becoming visible. It starts to stink and leak. Your partner is like, "What in the world is that? I didn't have any idea that came with you." And you think, *Um, how do we deal with this stuff? I wasn't expecting all this.*

That absolutely happened with us. Hope's depression was one big part of it. Me being an idiot was the other.

When I was growing up, probably because of my turned-up feeler and my learning issues, I think my mom felt a little sorry for me—especially when I hit junior high and kids were making fun of me, because both of my older brothers were very popular and good-looking. She became a short-order cook. I never balanced a checkbook in my life. I would bounce checks; she would take care of it. Anything and everything. You can imagine what I was like when Hope and I got married.

Here's just one example. I had been into sports all my life; I had played all sports, watched all sports, was a fan of all sports. Hope grew up the opposite way, believing that sports were silly and maybe even kind of bad, because there's always a loser. She did not like sports and did not get sports.

Shortly after we were married, I would use my Sunday afternoons just the way I grew up using them. I'd get my sweet tea and a bag of chips, go upstairs, and turn on the football game. Meanwhile, Hope would be slaving downstairs in the kitchen for two hours making this big, wonderful Sunday dinner, which is the way both of us grew up, and it's also kind of customary for the area we grew up in. When the noise of the pots and pans got loud, I'd shout, "Hey, honey, could you keep that down? I'm trying to watch the game."

When it was time for dinner, I would eat dinner in seven minutes, grab more sweet tea and chips, and go back to the ball game. She finished dinner herself and then started the hour of cleanup. I would usually ask her another time or two to please hold it down.

When she'd finished with the kitchen, she would start vacuuming. That really annoyed me because I couldn't hear anything over the vacuum cleaner, and I vividly remember saying, "Honey, can you please do that somewhere else or some other time? I'm trying to watch the game."

Now, when I think about that, it seems like that was another person. How in the world could I have ever been so stupid? To have that turned-up feeler and act that way is ridiculous, because if I had just taken thirty seconds to think, *What if I were Hope in this scenario?* I'd have been furious. That sort of thing just really never occurred to me because it's the way I grew up. I thought it was normal.

Slowly, me being an idiot and her being depressed put more and more pressure on everything. Little things turned into big things over the course of the next two years. One of them was my mother dying of liver cancer. Another was me getting us into a huge financial hole, because if I wanted something I bought it, and I was used to my parents taking care of it if I got in trouble.

By the time I was in my mid-twenties, I was constantly asking myself questions like:

- How do I feel better and have more energy?
  (I was exhausted all the time and was plagued with acid reflux and migraine headaches.)
- How do I make more money? (I was about to go bankrupt.)
- How do I get my wife to be nicer to me? (She didn't want to have sex with me often enough for me and seemed irritated with me a lot of the time.)
- How do I find a great career and not just suffer through a job I don't like for thirty years?

But the more I tried to pursue the answers, the worse everything got. I felt more and more stress, worse and worse physically and emotionally, and more and more distant from Hope. I spent money we didn't have on seminars, programs, and books, but it always ended up the same: I just couldn't do what they were asking me to do, or I did do it but did not see the promised results.

At first, I went where most people go: I'm the problem. Everyone else seems to be able to do well in all these areas. But I can't, so there must be something wrong with me. I already greatly suspected as much based on my problems growing up: not measuring up to my brother, almost flunking every single grade until graduate school, and being made fun of in the schoolyard for being short and fat. And regularly getting into trouble.

By the time we'd been married two years or so, we were both in a lot of pain. My mom had just died, and Hope's depression was at its worst. That was when Hope told me she wanted a divorce and asked me to leave. I did not want a divorce, but I was unhappy in the marriage, too. I had hit rock bottom.

I had lost my health, my finances, my peace of mind, and now my marriage.

Why couldn't I get myself to do what was best for me and the ones I loved?

THE CHEMISTRY OF RIGHT AND WRONG

There are at least two reasons why the Law of Externals makes it nearly impossible to do what's best in our lives, whether it relates to dating, marriage, parenting, health, addictions, career, finances, or whatever our biggest problem is. The first has to do with the chemistry of right and wrong.

Depending on their meaning, our memories trigger one of four chemical states:

1. *Fear.* If you do or even imagine something that your memories tell you is dangerous, your brain tells your hypothalamus to release cortisol, adrenaline, and dopamine—it's time to run, fight, or hide, and it leads to that whole list of negative results we've been referring to in the last few chapters.

2. *Neutral.* If you do or imagine something that does not trigger a danger memory, but also doesn't necessarily trigger a love-based memory, your brain tells the hypothalamus that it can ease off the reins, and we have reasonable access to our conscious mind and our conscience. The conscience, our love compass, is automatically activated when our life-or-death response is not. It contains the law of love and morality that is also programmed into the heart, and it helps us know how to choose love in any given situation. This is how our unconscious can help us do what we need to do.

3. *Love.* If you do or imagine something that triggers a love-based memory and does not trigger a fear-based memory, your brain tells the hypothalamus to ease off *and* releases chemicals that lead to love, joy, peace, power,

etc., leading to that list of positive results we've been referring to.

Now, there is a fourth situation that arises—this is when you're faced with a decision to do something that you know you shouldn't do, but that you very much want to do, whether it's eating ice cream or chocolate, having that second or third drink, binge watching a TV show, flirting when you're married, or stealing pens from work.

> 4. *Tidal wave.* If you do or imagine doing something pleasurable for an extended period *that you believe is wrong*, your brain tells your hypothalamus to release *all* the chemicals of both love and fear:
> ○ Dopamine
> ○ Norepinephrine
> ○ Oxytocin
> ○ Serotonin
> ○ Endorphins

This cascade is equivalent to a drug overdose, where you lose control of your actions. It is absolutely overwhelming and often leads to addiction.

Researchers discovered this phenomenon when studying Internet pornography. They noticed that when participants viewed pornography *and also believed it was wrong*, they experienced this chemical tidal wave. This didn't happen as strongly for people who viewed pornography and *didn't* believe it was wrong.[1]

It reminds me of a saying from the Bible: if you think something is wrong and do it, for you it is wrong.

To me this is an amazing statement. If you believe keeping a hundred-dollar bill you find on the sidewalk is wrong and you do it, your body has a chemical reaction on the same spectrum (although obviously much less heightened) as if you murdered someone. What ancient wisdom said is true, we now know based on chemistry.

But if we do something pleasurable we believe is wrong, we get *all* the chemicals. That's what creates the addiction. To continue the example of Internet porn, as a result of the tidal wave of chemicals released, the person feels physical and non-physical energy, desire, a form of fulfillment, and even something akin to love. However, typically after the moment of release, the feelings and thoughts almost immediately change to guilt, regret, self-loathing, etc. Very often the individual will then need to do something else to deal with these new problems. The reason they viewed the porn in the first place was to deal with a different set of problems: boredom, unfulfilled desire, stress release, etc. Then after the second set of problems diminishes, the first set typically returns. The result is a vicious cycle that keeps you trapped in a loop. You are now chemically dependent—on internal chemicals. And you also now have memories of particular people (those you watched) that have both love (good) and guilt (wrong) labels.

What's the result? You are overpowered, even if you are a strong person. Once you cross a line, you almost can't turn back. Once you imagine finally doing something you believe is wrong for you for a significant period of time, you're a puppet to your chemicals and electrical signals. This is far worse than just fear. The combination is so potent, once you get to a certain point, you almost can't resist—no one can. In my opinion, this is at the root of the sexual and physical harassment, and all the hatred and violence that we hear about daily. Good people who can't get themselves to do what they believe they should and who can't stop themselves from doing what they know that they shouldn't. And because we aren't aware of this internal chemical tidal wave trigger, we tend to blame it on our external circumstances and rationalize our choices.

I did the Hulk ride at Universal Studios many years ago, and, man, what a rush! But it wasn't even close to the chemical rush I would have had if I had been imagining doing something I believed was wrong for an extended period of time. Not just Internet pornography, of course, but anything I believed was pleasurable but wrong. For me, it could be having a Dr Pepper. For Hope, it could be eating chocolate. Whatever is on your personal list of guilty pleasures. The stronger your emotions around the event, the stronger the tidal wave.

This phenomenon typically happens when your brain is in the fear state—when you're living under the Law of Externals. You're in an unstable, painful place already, so you're looking for pleasure or a distraction—even when you know it's wrong. That doesn't mean that people living by the Law of Internals never do anything exciting or illicit; it's just that they don't experience the same tidal wave of stimulation that would likely then enforce the behavior and make it that much harder to avoid the next time. When fear is in control, your unconscious would rather have you choose wrong than choose pain, because our basic fear-based survival programming is to seek pleasure and avoid pain. And when you're living under the Law of Externals, especially if you're anything close to a perfectionist, think of how many things are considered "wrong"—and how many times a day you're activating this tidal wave of chemicals!

According to Daniel Amen, MD, reactivated memories result in the same chemical reaction as the original event, so you experience the same chemical release even when you simply imagine or remember doing that wrong but pleasurable thing.

In fact, before you do something wrong, you always imagine it first in your experience simulator in the prefrontal cortex. You imagine it as positive (or at least pleasurable), or you wouldn't do it. But your experience simulator is lying to you; as Dan Gilbert said, most of us are terrible predictors of what our experiences will be like! You know at the same time that it's wrong for you, which triggers the release of cortisol. You do it anyway because of the pleasurable image and the chemicals you are experiencing while you're imaging it. The addition of the cortisol, dopamine, and oxytocin magnifies the chemical experience, and you quickly reach a point of no return.

So you are in essence experiencing "wrong" and "good" at the same moment, which is what creates such an intense reaction. This chemical overdose can start to destroy the positive effects of oxytocin, even from your existing love memories, by assigning "love" tags to something that is actually wrong for you, thus literally changing your unconscious definition of love. If adrenaline is released during an event, it is tagged as a fear event. If oxytocin is released, it is labeled a love event.

Here's another example. When I was a kid, the TV show *Dallas* was huge. Every week was a new episode of lying, cheating, having affairs, plotting, and conniving. Today there are dozens of shows that would fit into that category. My mother was absolutely addicted to it. She could not miss an episode. Whenever anyone would ask her about it, she would say, "I know I shouldn't watch it, but I just have to see what that J.R. does next, and laugh!"

So every week, she retreated to her bedroom to watch *Dallas* by herself. As children, we were forbidden to watch it, and my dad was very strict and religious, so he wanted nothing to do with it. Even though we kids thought it was funny (my dad certainly didn't), my mother believed she shouldn't be watching it, and I can guarantee she was experiencing that tidal wave every week, which kept her in that addictive cycle.

The research says it's your belief about it that matters. So my advice is, if you decide to have a half gallon of ice cream, enjoy every spoonful! Some of the most unhealthy people I've ever seen are people who are so controlled that they never treat themselves, which can be like putting a lid on a boiling pot. Of course, try to keep in balance overall. The bottom line: try to live what you believe is right, and when you slip up, make it right with God and others, and forgive yourself.

However, this is very difficult if you are in the Law of Externals system. Not only is your list of things that are "wrong" extremely long, you're also constantly in a state of fear, which means you're programmed to prioritize seeking pleasure and avoiding pain over your considerations of right and wrong.

How many times a day do you do what you believe is wrong because it's pleasurable and release this chemical overdose into your system? How can you possibly choose what is best for you in this scenario? You're set up for failure every time!

A STATE OF SHOCK

In addition to the constant chemical overdose we receive by consistently doing something momentarily pleasurable and wrong, choosing the Law of Externals also results in losing access to the parts of our brain that know what's best for us to begin with.

First of all, when we choose the fear-based Law of Externals, we have essentially put ourselves in a constant state of survival mode. Our brain knows that our unconscious is much better equipped to help us survive than our conscious willpower. The difference in speed between our unconscious and our conscious is like the difference between today's supercomputer and the first-generation computer from the 1950s. In other words, if survival is our goal, trying to survive with our conscious free will is suicide. We'll get ourselves hurt, and maybe killed. You literally don't have time to avoid almost any close-call car wreck if you are limited to your conscious mind's response time. Fortunately, in these situations, your unconscious forcibly takes over, bypasses your conscious mind, and puts your foot on the brake before you have time to think about it.

For better or worse, our programming won't let us deal with these situations consciously. This is great when it's a car wreck—it saves your life. But when everything in our life is driven by fear, the unconscious becomes our best driver. So when we choose the Law of Externals, our unconscious mind puts the survival part of our mind in the driver's seat and mandates fear-based thoughts, feelings, behaviors, and brain chemistry. We've lost easy access to our conscience and a large portion of our conscious mind. In other words, your unconscious says, "Get out of the driver's seat and go sit over there; we've got this."

The best analogy I can think of is being in a state of shock. Let's say Linda was in a car wreck. She's got a cut on her head and a few scratches on her arms. Outside of that, she's unharmed, but the car is totaled. She's sitting there on the side of the road, and the paramedic comes and starts talking to her, but she doesn't respond at all.

The paramedic, because he's trained, says, "Linda? Linda? Linda? Is your name Linda? Do you live in Michigan? Is your husband's name Tom?" He claps his hands in front of her eyes. Maybe he gives her some smelling salts. He says, "Okay, Linda, you are in shock. You're okay. We're going to take care of you."

Well, what's the deal there? The deal is, Linda's gone. Her unconscious survival mind has taken over, and in this case, it's just taken her away. She's hiding internally. Not because she chose to, but because the unconscious commanded it.

That's an extreme form of what the mind does constantly in me and in you every day. Based on the pain we experience and the choice we've made about the system of right and wrong that we've chosen and are going to live by, the unconscious takes over and feeds us its own constructs. It may work short-term, but very often it's harmful in the long term. You don't have access to your highest abilities in your conscience and conscious mind, because your unconscious is focused on physical survival.

So that's what the unconscious does when you end up in the Law of Externals—it keeps you alive, even if the way it does that isn't the best for you, and even if it has to deceive you to do it.

Here's the bottom line: as a result of the memory malfunction we've been describing for the past few chapters, most people on most days are effectively in a mild state of shock, and your unconscious mind has taken partial control away from your conscious mind. Now, rather than experiencing things as they are, your experiences are filtered through an overly vigilant lens that would rather be overly protected than overly vulnerable. And the thoughts and feelings it mandates are always negative.

Even worse, your survival mind has tricked you into believing you do have control, so you believe these choices are actually yours and entirely justified. Effectively, you're spending a great deal of energy constantly rationalizing why you believe the earth is really flat after all.

So what if, when you're in this state, you want to go on a new diet and get in better shape? SORRY! Start a new career path to do what you love or be more successful? NOPE! Turn over a new leaf and start prioritizing healthy relationships so you can experience more love, joy, and peace in your life? NOT GONNA HAPPEN! Just fill in the blank with whatever major, positive, lasting changes you want to make—WRONG ANSWER, THANKS FOR PLAYING! At least long term.

Why? Because each of those decisions will require short-term pain and discomfort for long-term gain. All positive growth does. But that's something the survival brain is not capable of doing. It runs on the programming of pain equals danger equals death. Pleasure equals good equals happiness. But it's a lie. Eventually, your unconscious is going to decide the temporary pain associated with a diet, or a new exercise routine, or the learning curve of a new job is "killing" you, and command you to eat the bag of cookies, watch some mindless TV, go back to the dead-end job, or take on too much work again. It will direct you to something that is short-term pleasurable or lessens pain, which more often than not takes you into a vicious cycle (habit or addiction).

But please hear this loud and clear: *it's not your fault!* Your unconscious mind has taken over your decision-making because of a memory malfunction in your brain and nervous system that has evolved over thousands of years and that scientists have only recently discovered. You were born with it. We all were. And it's getting worse with every generation.

Here's the great irony: the fact that we can't consistently do what's best wouldn't bother us so much if we lived in the grace system! It only bothers us because we've chosen the survival system!

Approximately 3 percent of people can live by what they believe is right and best on their own. For whatever reason, they don't have the unconscious "junk" that most of the rest of us have. If you are in that group, you know it. You tend to think and act positively, and when you want to change something, it isn't difficult for you to do it. You bounce back from pain quickly and are most likely successful (in your own way).

As for the rest of us, we have lost the ability to consistently do what we know is best and forgive ourselves when we don't, no matter how hard we try.

THE ILLUSION OF FREE WILL

This is pretty much what researchers have been saying for the last several decades, but no one's been paying much attention to them because I don't think anyone really wants to believe it. Just recently, The Atlantic published an article about the implications of this research, titled, "There's No Such Thing as Free Will."[2] It chronicled the research beginning in the nineteenth century, and especially in the last several decades, that has determined that our actions are not the result of our free, conscious choice, but of subconscious and unconscious brain activity.

When the researchers say you don't have the free will to choose your thoughts, feelings, and actions, what they're ultimately saying is that you don't have the ability to choose the most successful, happiest, and best course for yourself, and for those you love and care about. You are, in essence, almost like a wooden puppet that believes it's a real person!

One of the researchers interviewed in the Atlantic article stated that even though the evidence is unequivocal, it might be best if nobody knew about it. If you know anything about science and researchers, you know how ridiculous that statement sounds. "Not tell anyone about my breakthrough discovery, my life's work—are you *out of your mind?*!"

Why would they want to hide it? Because—at least as far as the researchers know—there's nothing you can do about it, and based on further studies, they also know that if you thought you didn't have the free will to change your life, it would greatly diminish your happiness and satisfaction, and maybe even cause you to give up.

Yet the idea of the illusion of free will is far from new: *National Geographic's Your Brain: A User's Guide* (2012) calls it the "illusion of intention," citing research that shows an electrical spike in the unconscious mind sets actions in motion before any activity occurs in the conscious mind.[3] Other studies have identified the significant role that the vagus nerve—controlled by our unconscious—has on our thoughts, emotions, and behaviors.[4]

Once I asked William Tiller, PhD, what he believed was most important, based on his decades of research and lab testing. He said, "Intention." I asked him if he believed in unconscious intention as well as conscious intention. His response was, "Absolutely, and typically your conscious intention doesn't work until you fix the unconscious intention that is limiting you."

Many centuries ago, manuscripts of ancient wisdom described the same phenomenon in different language: "I do not do the good I want, but the evil I do not want is what I keep doing."[5] That's from the Apostle Paul, one of the most famous religious figures in history. I had lunch with a friend the other day, and he said to me, "Why is it that I keep doing what I don't want to do, and can't do what I want to do?" Most of us are still asking that question today.

To a different degree, it's also what bestselling author

Stephen R. Covey called "the tyranny of the urgent"—it's why we have so much trouble prioritizing what we know is ultimately most important. We've all experienced the simple fact that we do not have full control over our thoughts, feelings, and actions. It's been going on for a long, long time. It's just that science has only recently been able to explain how it happens.

So, if all this is true, what do the researchers suggest we do? Well, the ones who believe it's best to hide the truth are basically saying we should placebo ourselves—just keep believing the illusion that our conscious mind and conscious intention are in charge of our actions (even though science says otherwise), so we don't completely self-destruct as we live our compromised, malfunctioning life! In other words, we should believe and live a lie, because it's the best we can do. That's what "placebo" effectively means in this case: to believe something that isn't true. And that's exactly what most personal development authors and experts tell us to do (whether they realize it or not). They tell us that to live a life of meaning and purpose, all we have to do is decide what we believe is most meaningful, make a plan to live that way, and then use our conscious mind and our willpower to follow the plan. They're asking us to believe the lie that our conscious mind is stronger than our unconscious and that we can take control over our thoughts, feelings, and actions. If you remember *The Matrix*, it's like they're asking us to just take another blue pill and stay in the world of illusion!

Our other choice, according to the experts, is to greatly reduce our definition of free will, accept that our unconscious runs our lives much like other mammals, and make the most of the limited free will we do have.[6] Like animals, we can't change the fact that we're primarily living to seek pleasure and avoid pain, according to the Law of Externals. We just need to make the most of living in survival mode. That's why some experts have started focusing on helping us adjust to stress or find its positive effects.[7] And some studies have found that what we believe about stress—our stress mind-set—can positively counteract some of its negative effects.

This sounds like great news—but again, it's actually old news. These studies are simply further proving the placebo effect. The placebo effect, or the power of whether we believe something will work (or not), has been well known for decades. When you believe something will have a positive effect on you, its real positive effect increases significantly for about 30 percent of people, but typically only for a short time. In other words, it has a limited positive effect for a limited amount of time. The only thing that's different is science's mind-set about the placebo effect: some scientists are beginning to spin it positively rather than as an embarrassment they couldn't explain!

What hasn't changed is the negative effect stress has on us. What researchers call the positive effects of stress, resulting when stress is viewed from a positive mind-set, are simply a biochemical combination of positive belief (placebo) plus the negative presence of stress. For example, stress may cause you to get more done, and therefore get a raise and all the things that come with more money. This may be true for a short time period, but you still have all the negative effects of stress as well—cortisol overdose and crash, suppressed immune system, feeling dumbed down, reduced creativity, etc. If that weren't enough, recent research has shown that cortisol has also been linked to brain shrinkage and memory problems.[8]

If you want real, lasting relief from stress, you'd have to ask: why settle for a limited positive effect over a limited amount of time? The positive chemicals of love give you all the positive results without any of the negative. Why not greatly reduce or remove the stress completely and experience full, long-term transformation, so that your life keeps getting better and better? Why not get rid of the source of stress to begin with—especially if it's based on an internal lie in the first place?

I believe these researchers have done some wonderful work and are truly trying to help people. I also think they're focusing on making the best of it because they assume the source of stress can't be removed. But it can. The difference between a life of placebo, where a little internal love and truth is mixed in with a lot of internal fear and falsehood, and a life spent in love and truth as the default is like the difference between a candle and the sun.

What I've been describing as the great memory malfunction is why many experts say "people don't change." I disagree with this statement, but I am in a tiny minority. Changing negative patterns long term no longer has to be rare. Rather than the 90 percent failure rate we've had in the past, I believe that we can have a 90 percent success rate. But before I show you how you can conquer these destructive internal patterns, let's summarize where we've been so far.

CHAPTER SIX

A Summary of the Great Memory Malfunction

We've covered a lot of material so far, and I know that some of it can be pretty overwhelming. But I hope that you're also finding at least some of this to be a relief. You are designed to live a life of love, joy, and peace, and you already have everything you need inside you to create it. If you've been consistently having trouble doing what you know is best in any area of your life, now you know it's because of the great memory malfunction I've been describing throughout part 1.

As a result of this malfunction, when your heart (which includes the unconscious, subconscious, conscious spirit, and right brain) is interpreting data through the lens of your memories, I believe it goes through something like a flow chart of these three questions. But remember, it's not searching for the truth, it's searching for your memories' internal definitions of the truth, which very well may be untrue. Here are the questions:

1. *Are you safe or in danger?* It's not just a matter of
   whether you're safe or not, it's whether you
   feel safe or not—physically or non-physically.
   If you sense that you're in danger, nothing
   else matters; your heart starts pushing certain
   buttons so you lose access to your prefrontal
   cortex and your conscience, your survival
   mechanism takes over, and you're flooded
   with the chemistry of fear. End of story.
      If you're safe, your brain moves to the next
   question.
2. *Which law are you following?* If it's the Law of
   Externals, your thoughts, feelings, brain
   chemistry, everything have the sole intention of
   keeping you alive physically and as comfortable
   as you can be. Doing the right thing for you,
   personally, is now a matter of life or death. It
   pushes the button to enact simple stimulus/
   response reward and punishment. Then, if
   you do something you believe is right, you
   may feel false pride, or just that you avoided
   punishment. Do something you believe is
   wrong, and it starts pushing a whole new series
   of buttons: the guilt button, the shame button,
   the insignificance button, and the double-life
   button. Then it goes to the next question.
3. *Who are you?* If your previous answer was the
   Law of Externals, your heart starts pushing
   the associated identity buttons, like "You are
   valuable based on what you do and don't do,

what you have and don't have." If you lived according to this law, you would seldom believe you were gifted and one of a kind and had a lot to offer the world (or if you did, it would be accompanied with arrogance). You would be caught in the cycle of superiority and inferiority, judging yourself based on how you compare to others around you.

If your answer to question one was that you are safe, and question two was the Law of Internals, your heart pushes buttons based on your true identity, like, "You are a good person! You have a talent. You are valuable. You have everything you really need. You are one of a kind." You can do what you need to do in life and fully savor your experiences. You can recover when painful things happen. You can trust and believe that things will work out for the best. (Questions one and two typically go together—both positive or both negative.)

Then, after it goes through that flow chart of three questions, your heart starts applying the law you've chosen to your current situation. If you've chosen the Law of Externals, your heart says, "Okay, your choice," and starts mandating fear, and all the things that go with it. We get to choose the law, but once we do, the system determines the experience, unless or until we make a different choice. The first button it pushes is stress, because you've got to do everything perfectly to be okay, or you have already given up on trying to do things right because you have tried many times and you can't (this was mine). The purpose of stress is to keep you physically alive for another day.

If you chose the Law of Internals, your heart pushes totally different buttons. It would ask, "Okay, in this situation, how can you enjoy doing something even if it used to be unpleasant? What is the right thing to do now? How can you prioritize relationships in this situation? How can you do whatever you are doing from a place of love for the next thirty minutes? What can you do to change the world for the better, change your family for the better, be the best you can be, and become happy?"

That stuff wouldn't even be on the radar screen for your unconscious if you chose the external system! Now, it might be on your *conscious* radar screen—it may be all your conscious mind thinks about. But your unconscious is going to be constantly working against your best intentions, which is why you struggle to sustainably do what's best for you in the important areas of your life, and why you keep doing what you know isn't best for you.

Your heart goes through that three-step sequence in a nanosecond whenever it's faced with a new experience, and with every new day. Most people get stuck on number one, because they have so many errors in their memories and never feel completely safe. But even if you get past that one, the second one usually gets you, because the great majority of people are governed by the wrong law, usually thinking it is the only law.

In terms of our internal state and our body chemistry, this memory malfunction is akin to what it would be like if the local fire department showed up at your house every time you turned on your stove! So every time you started to cook dinner, firefighters would show up with sirens blaring to get everyone out of the house!

Now, if that happened in our home, would we stop cooking and avoid the stove at all costs? Would we buy ear protection for ourselves and our family and use the stove as much as we could tolerate (but despite our best efforts, find ourselves ordering takeout far more than was good for us)? Would we meditate for hours each morning so the ear-splitting noise didn't bother us so much? No! We'd think, *Gosh, the fire alarm is seriously malfunctioning,* and we'd get it fixed or replace it. The only way we'd mess with any of that other stuff was if we thought the smoke alarm couldn't be fixed.

That's exactly what's happening with our life-or-death survival response. It's clearly malfunctioning, but we don't respond in a way that gets us any closer to getting it fixed. We just assume that we feel the way we do because our broken alarms can't be fixed, or that our constant stress is normal. We just try to get through each day as best we can rather than pausing to figure out whether a better way might be possible.

We exercise like crazy, take supplements, and eat ultra-clean food to help counteract the negative effects the long-term release of cortisol is having on our bodies. Or we give up. We meditate for hours a day to find some relief from our stress-crazed thoughts and feelings. We may also choose to drink, take drugs, or engage in extreme (but unhealthy) behaviors that supply a rush of pleasure for a short period of time. And all to cope with something that should never be coped with—it *has* to be fixed, like the fire alarm or the water spewing onto the floor!

We feel disconnected from our meaning and purpose because our actions are governed by fight-or-flight: we're either running from the pain of our malfunctioning internal fire alarm or we're seeking any pleasure that can temporarily allow us to escape it.

Think back to how we were created to live, with our internal fear alarm going off only during true emergencies. If we had grown up living primarily in love, joy, and peace, looking forward to whatever the day held, and then out of the blue everyone's internal fire alarm started malfunctioning the way it is right now, there would be a worldwide panic! We'd consider it one of the worst pandemics to hit the human race, because we'd all remember what it was like to have our conscious mind and our conscience in positive harmony with the unconscious, and the positive actions that naturally flow from that most of the time. But because this memory malfunction has happened gradually over thousands of years—like the frog in a pot of slowly heating water who never realizes he's being boiled to death—we all think it's normal, because everyone around us is living this way, too. But the tragedy of how far we've fallen is the same.

Only at the end of our lives do we find ourselves looking back and thinking, *How did I end up here? If I could just have another go at my life...*

There is another way.

In chapter 1, I mentioned that the left brain has a

very important function. Here it is. The most important function of your left brain is to allow you at any time to choose to commit to the Law of Internals.

This is the most important choice. If you get this, you get everything.

Regardless of how you've lived to this point, today you still have the choice between prioritizing what's in it for me and what feels good in the moment, or fully committing to love, regardless of the pain, pleasure, or end results.

What does that choice mean? It means, "Even if I don't get pleasure and get even more pain, I am committed to love in the present moment as best I can, come what may. I am all in, nothing held back, no plan B, no safety net, forever, whether I get what I want or not."

Before a rocket takes off, it's locked down by mechanisms that keep it from accidentally taking off before everything is ready. Once the countdown begins, and mission control gets to zero, the safety features are released and the rocket blasts off, just as it was designed to do.

Your life is like that rocket, and your heart's safety features are keeping your life locked down. You need to be locked down until your conscious mind is developed enough to really choose between the Law of Internals and the Law of Externals. You can't get killed sitting safely in the rocket on the ground, but you may very well get killed hurtling thousands of miles an hour through the air; that's why your heart is inclined to keep your rocket grounded unless it trusts that the flight plan is a sound one—that's when you're able to lift off and soar.

In order to commit to the Law of Internals, I have

to give up the end result. Which end result? *All of them.* Will I be loved or hated? Will I be rich or poor? Popular or unpopular? Good health or chronic pain? Will people like me or not? Will I have to work hard or have it easy? I have to give up controlling all end results. Trying to control those results are not my job anymore. Those are love's jobs now, and love is a million times more powerful than I am. From my clients who have made this choice, I've heard it all: *Wow, my cancer went away! I'm making more money than I ever dreamed of. How did that happen?*

Here's my opinion of how it happens. I believe that the purpose of this life is to choose love over fear. That's it. Will I choose love or fear? It is my choice. Every day when I wake up, it's another opportunity to accomplish what my whole life is about. Another day that I have the opportunity to choose love rather than fear.

Your heart constantly looks to see which you will choose.

Here's how I believe your heart sees it. It knows the energy of love is a million times more powerful than your conscious effort alone. For that reason, love is the only thing more important than physical survival. Until you choose to prioritize love no matter what, avoiding death is the only thing that matters, because, hopefully, you'll live another day and have another opportunity to choose love. When you do, death is not the most important thing anymore; it's secondary. And that's when everything changes.

If you make that choice on your own, here's what your heart does. It announces, "*Attention!* She just got it! Remove the safety features! Let her fly!"

When we make that commitment to the Law of Internals, to do our best to live in love this moment regardless of end results, our safety features are released, and our life achieves liftoff.

Why? It's safe now. You've finally realized what's most important in life, and your heart knows it.

You win life!

When you do this, you regain access to your best resources—your conscience together with your conscious mind—and they start to do what they were made to do: produce seemingly miraculous results that are always win-win-win.

Here's how it happened for me. After Hope threw me out of the house, I threw everything overboard. I said to God, *I don't even know if you exist anymore.* I started reading every religious text I could get my hands on and asking others who had studied them for decades what they taught. I sought out wise people and asked them endless questions. I started praying and meditating like never before.

That led me to the most profound spiritual turnaround of my life, which I also wrote about in *The Love Code*. Late one night, I felt like God told me (as a thought in my head, not an audible voice), "Not only do you not love Hope, you don't even know what love is."

That was all I heard. I wanted more, but that was all I got.

So I went to the library and looked up the definition of love in every dictionary, textbook, and religious text I could find. I talked to religious leaders, people I respected—even a lawyer I knew.

Eventually I came to believe that the voice was right. I saw how I was all about sex for me, food for me, fun for me, while Hope did everything to provide that for me. I came to believe that love meant being all in with my relationships, no matter what.

I wasn't remotely living that way. I was living in a business deal. To truly love Hope, I would need to give up control.

And that's when I met Larry Napier, the man who would become my spiritual mentor from that moment on, and who started teaching me about the two laws.

I had night sweats and terrible nightmares because the Law of Externals was so ingrained in me. It was so strong. It had its tentacles in every part of my being. It felt almost like an exorcism.

I had believed all my life that the Law of Externals was the only law. It wasn't a choice; it was reality. To live a successful life, you've got to figure out how to do it right, make a plan, and work harder and harder to make that plan work. I kept thinking, *This law is not negotiable. Saying I can choose the Law of Internals is like saying I choose that the earth is flat. You can choose some things, but you can't choose that!*

Well, after about six weeks I came to know—not believe, but also really know—that the law Larry had been teaching me was real, and I consciously chose it.

It happened one night when I felt like God asked me, now that I knew what love really was—with no safety net, no plan B, and nothing held back—would I choose to love Hope now, even if nothing in our relationship changed? I didn't answer right away. At that time, she wanted a divorce. This meant choosing love could mean loving her if she married someone else and had children with another man. Was I really willing to do that?

But finally, after a few days of thinking and praying, I was able to decide. Yes, I would love Hope in that way. All in. No strings attached, forever. And I meant it from the bottom of my heart.

That's the choice my heart was waiting for. That's when I shifted out of shock and gained access to my conscience and full conscious mind to not only know what was best, but to have the power to actually do it.

That's also when the self-destructive life vow I had made as a kid was overwritten. It was like someone took out one software program and put in a different one. It took no effort of my own at all. It was almost like I was observing myself in the third person and thinking, *Wow, how did that happen?*

One of the coolest things that happens when you commit to love is that your heart, for the first time, deprioritizes your erroneous, fear-based memories and prioritizes your love-based memories. I felt like a kid again, experiencing love and happiness like I did before school started—but as a reasoning adult.

About six weeks after she had kicked me out of the house, Hope and I started dating again. She told me later that from the first moment she saw me she knew I was a changed man. We had a recommitment ceremony, in love more than we ever had been, which is the way it's been ever since is. I loved her with a passion I had never felt in my life, and she felt the same way about me. We were hugging and kissing all the time. It was absolutely wonderful.

After going through all that, I was sure I had the magic bullet and excitedly taught this to all my clients—and guess what? Not a single one of them could do it.

Why? They were trying to do it with their willpower, still taking control of the results. In other words, they were trying to commit to love by the rules of the Law of Externals, which would never work.

That's when I realized this instant override doesn't happen with everyone. Over the next several years, I came up with a step-by-step memory engineering process that did work for nearly every one of my clients.

Why did I experience this kind of spontaneous shift, while many of my clients needed a more mechanical process to change their memories?

I believe it's because I hit bottom. In fact, many people I've talked to have a spontaneous shift like this when they also hit bottom in life. However, if I had had access to this kind of mechanical process earlier, maybe I wouldn't have had to hit bottom in the first place.

That's what I've seen with my clients: when they use the Memory Engineering Technique, they can change dramatically without having to hit bottom.

And that's why I wrote this book: so you don't have to hit bottom. Because I've seen a whole lot of clients get their free will back, heal their memories, and live the extraordinary life their hearts, minds, bodies, and spirits were meant to live.

Your constant stress response may be common today, but it's not normal. It's a malfunction, but the malfunction can be fixed—which is what you'll learn to do in part 2.

PART TWO

The Memory Engineering Technique

CHAPTER SEVEN

Energy Medicine 101

Before we get to the nuts and bolts of the Memory Engineering Technique, we need to cover two foundational concepts: *energy medicine* and *memory engineering*.

One day, when I was having lunch with my friend Dr. William Tiller, former head of the physics department at Stanford, I asked him a question.

"All my life I've heard about Einstein's famous equation, E equals mc squared, but I still don't understand it. What does that really mean?"

"Well, Alex," he said, "it's really very simple. On one side of the equation is energy, and on the other side is everything else." Everything in the universe boils down to energy. Dr. Tiller's rather famous quote, based on his work at Stanford, is "Future medicine will be based on controlling energy in the body."

Energy medicine is based on the recognition that everything is made of energy. Beneath everything we can sense and measure, there's an underlying energy pattern creating it that has a particular energy frequency. That includes not just our physical bodies, but our thoughts, feelings, and experiences as well. Energy medicine simply means using, adjusting, and changing the energy at the root of any human problem—whether it's emotional, intellectual, physical, spiritual, or all of those—to create a positive effect.

Nobel Prize winner Albert Szent-Györgyi, MD, PhD, said, "In every culture before ours, healing was accomplished by moving energy in the person's body." That may be hard to believe, but it is absolutely true. The field of energy medicine traces back to at least 1,500 BC.

You might be thinking, *Okay. If that's true, then how come I've never heard of it? Where did it go?* First of all, you have heard of it, but you might not call it energy medicine. CT scans, MRIs, lithotripsy for kidney stones, yoga, tai chi, acupuncture, Reiki, and even some forms of meditation are all energy medicine techniques.

It's also true that energy medicine (which includes what many refer to as energy psychology) has been making a tidal-wave resurgence over the last twenty years. The Healing Codes are an energy medicine technique, and when I wrote my first book on them back in 2001, energy medicine was about as far from mainstream as you could get. In 2007, Dr. Oz predicted that energy medicine would be the next big frontier in medicine. I believe his prediction is coming true right now. In fact, I'm told it's the fastest growing area in all of health. Why? Three reasons: it works, it's cheap, and there are no side effects.

My city of Nashville is a good example. When I started the Healing Codes, we were working out of my basement. At first, when I told people in Nashville what I did, they would say something like, "Oh, that's interesting," and then quickly change the subject. Around that same time, when I shared what I did with people in California, Europe, and Asia, they would say, "Oh, that's really cool. How can I find out more about that?"

Today, we have clients in all fifty states and 172 countries, virtually all from word of mouth. Now when I share with people in Nashville what I do, their response has been, "Oh, wow. That's really cool. How can I find more about that?" The times, they are a-changin'!

I recently had a conversation with a group of millennials (the age group of both my sons). To my amazement, they were telling me that in their age group, "energy" is a part of their daily conversations. It's not so much "pray for me" or "send me some love" as it is "send me some good energy." They said just about everyone they knew viewed energy healing and energy work as very positive and accepted. I thought, *How cool!* I had no idea it was that prevalent among the younger age groups.

Energy medicine is becoming more mainstream every day. The American Psychological Association recently approved the Association for Comprehensive Energy Psychology to sponsor continuing education credits, and experts also believe that approval for using these techniques in professional practice, with insurance coverage, is imminent. At a recent NBA final, I saw that professional basketball players had their own acupuncturists and other energy specialists. You regularly see people wearing energy bands on their arms. Energy medicine is positively affecting people around the world today, and it has been for thousands of years.

A WORD ABOUT DOUBLE-BLIND STUDIES

Even though energy medicine has been used around the world for thousands of years, even though people are being helped by energy medicine every day often when nothing else works, and even though more and more studies are showing its effectiveness, some people still automatically resist learning more about energy medicine because there aren't enough double-blind scientific studies "proving" it.

Earlier in the book, I told you what I think about double-blind studies. I'd like to take a minute to briefly review how double-blind studies became the supposed gold standard of scientific study. It all began with the plagues and smallpox pandemics, when thousands and even millions of people were dying and no one could do anything about it. Then they discovered a vaccination—a chemical—could stop it.

Before that, as Albert Szent-Györgyi said, healing was accomplished largely by natural substances and by changing energy. So why did we throw out natural, energy-based medicine when it had worked so well for centuries—to the point that today it seems strange, fringe, and woo-woo?

I believe it was a result of fear. It makes sense: when those horrible things were happening, everyone was reacting out of fear and panic. Everyone was afraid that their family was going to get the black plague, or their child was going to get smallpox. All of a sudden, the field of medicine focused entirely on testing chemicals to treat disease. Over time, pharmaceuticals completely replaced energy medicine as the standard of care. And the double-blind study became the gold standard for making sure that the chemical did what it was supposed to do and its benefits outweighed its negative side effects.

I believe those vaccinations were wonderful, life-saving discoveries. There's a place for them when your life is truly in danger. But as a field of study, I believe we've thrown the baby out with the bathwater. We've gone too far out of balance, and we forgot that natural, energy-based medicine worked pretty well for probably thousands of years, and few people got hurt or killed by it.

With the tidal-wave resurgence of energy medicine, I believe we are moving in a positive direction of greater balance.

Again, I am not against the scientific method, double-blind studies, or standard medicine. But for many things in the natural and energy health field, there are no medical tests for what is being treated. Show me the medical test that measures whether my memory of my dad hitting me has had the low self-worth removed from it. It doesn't exist.

So rather than only looking for a double-blind study to prove something, I also look to other sources for evidence of the truth that is not yet proven:

1. *Ancient texts.* Ancient religious and philosophical texts are filled with wisdom; we just haven't been able to prove a lot of it yet. So I begin by asking, "What do the ancients say?" Those men and women didn't have smartphones, the TV, or the Internet. They sat around together for hours a day and talked about the issues of their day all the time. Their scientists

and medical experts weren't only looking at chemicals; in fact, they didn't have access to the majority of the drugs that we have today. They did the best that they could by looking at how the mind worked and how the natural resources that they had available could be used to heal and alleviate pain in the patient.

2. *Credible scientific and/or anecdotal evidence.* Here I rely on Jimmy Netterville's advice: if it doesn't do harm, and it works pretty consistently— go for it! When people experience a lasting improvement or a true relief from suffering, it's important to look at what they did, even if we don't understand fully how it works. And tell me about it, so I can refer my people to it.

3. *Resonance with my heart.* I need to take a bit more time to explain this one. Dr. Lipton calls this experience of resonance a "vibe" that is almost always right. It's what happens the split-second before your foot slams on the brake to avoid an accident: your body perceives information that your conscious mind isn't aware of, your brain sends an electrical signal telling the right leg to take your foot off the gas and put it on the brake, and you avoid hitting the stopped car in front of you, before you're even aware of what's happening. In fact, this happens whenever we make a decision: as the research on conscious intention showed, one second before we

consciously make a decision, there's an electrical spike in our brain. Our heart had already perceived and processed an immense amount of data before our conscious mind ever got involved and sent that electrical signal to tell the conscious mind what it should do. I believe that the body does this not only in the extreme situations, like the avoided car accident, but also when it comes to modalities of healing.

Early in my career, I studied with Savely Yurkovsky, MD, who developed a technique called Field Control Therapy. Dr. Yurkovsky taught that there is an invisible "pilot" of every cell connected to the pilots of every other cell that exists, otherwise known as the *super-quantum*. They are somehow able to communicate with each other in such a way that the cell will act in an unpredictable way to save itself. I believe this phenomenon is behind the true stories we hear about people knowing things they can't possibly know, what Einstein called "action at a distance," and what some people call ESP. The fact that all cells are connected in some way is not a new idea. Most ancient religions and spiritualities would call this "spirit." For example, there's a quote from the Bible that says, "the Spirit himself testifies with our spirit that we are children of God."[1] If you read the full context,

you'll see that it means, "I know something
I have no way of knowing, and the source of
that I'm calling Spirit."

I believe what Dr. Yurkovsky called the
super-quantum is another way of describing
what Bruce Lipton calls "vibe," what ancient
religions and spiritualities called "spirit,"
what many today might call "intuition," what
Einstein called "spooky action at a distance,"
and what I'm calling "resonance." I believe
that we can train ourselves to listen closely
to that resonance; when we do, we gain the
ability to tell when we're on the right track.

4. *Results.* What actually happens when I try
   it? Does anything change for the better,
   consistently, when it is done? Does anything
   change for the worse?

5. *Prayer.* This is the most important source of
   evidence for me. I talk or "plug in" to a higher
   power to express my desire—for healing, for
   clarity, for peace, for guidance. I call that power
   God; others may refer to it as Source, Buddha,
   Allah, Spirit, or your Higher Power. Some also
   talk about accessing your intuition or your
   conscience, but to me this is different from
   plugging into the spiritual higher power, where
   miracles are possible. When you ask from a
   place of calm, and listen with a clear mind, you
   will be astonished by the answers you receive.

When all five of these things line up in the same direction, I have *never* found it to be wrong or damaging. Ever.

If you're looking for definitive, 100 percent empirical proof of energy medicine from double-blind studies, you're out of luck. There are no tests that currently can measure what it does or even the part of us that it's working in. Does energy medicine work for every person every time? No, but nothing does. My wife was depressed for twelve years, and everything the doctor recommended, based on clinical studies, did not work. None of the so-called miracle drugs they tried worked.

As I said at the beginning of the book, you and your family can benefit from energy medicine in twenty years once we're able to prove it, or you can benefit from it now.

The reason it's not part of mainstream medicine right now is that we aren't able to reliably measure the energy patterns of the unconscious mind yet, but that's just because we haven't developed the right technology. As Dr. Oz said, "We're beginning now to understand things we know in our hearts are true but could never measure."

Why does he say "things we know in our hearts are true"? Nine out of ten people who try the proven energy medicine techniques—like the Memory Engineering Technique you'll learn in this book—feel the difference. Most people "feel" the Memory Engineering Technique working in about ten minutes. They know in their heart it's working.

But you won't be able to experience this just by reading

about it. You have to do it. It's the difference between reading the words "glass of water" on a piece of paper and drinking a glass of water. Or the difference between seeing a picture of the Grand Canyon and seeing it in person.

You cannot experience the Grand Canyon to the fullest extent from a picture. It's absolutely impossible. Now, you can experience a little bit of it, you can get a sense of how it will impact you, but I promise you it is nothing like what you feel when you step up to that observation point for the first time in your life, and you see the sun shining on those cliffs and the Colorado River running through the middle. There is no way you can get that from a picture. Energy medicine and energy psychology have become a tidal wave because of people's *experience*, and there's no way you can evaluate that without sharing it.

So, feel free to Google it and do all the research you want to do, but understand that as Dr. Oz said, we really don't have devices that can go far enough and deep enough to measure these things yet. But your heart will tell you if it's working.

ENERGY MEDICINE RESEARCH

All that is not to say we don't have scientific evidence for energy medicine. In part 1, we mentioned Dr. Bruce Lipton's research at Stanford that showed thoughts, feelings, and beliefs (what he called the "environment" of a cell) change physiology.[2] Thoughts, feelings, and beliefs are forms of energy, and that energy made verifiable changes at the cellular level.

The studies done to verify that changing energy changes physiology are too numerous to cite here.[3] But I will cite one study done just recently. Our company, the Healing Codes, had a contact at a water company with very sophisticated and expensive water testing equipment. We wanted them to help us do a test to see if a non-physical energy frequency would manifest itself in any measurable way in the physical realm. They did independent testing on the effect a particular harmonic frequency had upon the physiology of water. Specifically, they were asked to test for copper, because the FDA has recently approved copper for killing microbes that cause the MRSA virus and staph infections. Now hospitals are putting copper strips on countertops, for example, to reduce infections.

The water company began with a sealed bottle of Dasani water that, when opened and tested, had 0 parts per million of copper before the experiment. A harmonic-frequency-generating device, tuned to the harmonic frequency of copper, was then put beside the water. The second test showed a copper reading of 2 parts per million. Water experts recommend a level of 0.5 to 1.5 parts copper per million in pools to eliminate algae, so a 2 was a very significant amount and more than was needed to rid the water of harmful microbes. The water company expert described the test as "weird" and "a little mind blowing." In fact, he said, "This is impossible."

Note that the water testing equipment does not test for the harmonic frequency of anything—it tests only for the actual, physical presence of copper. The conclusion was that the harmonic frequency produced physical copper in the water. This drove the technician so crazy that he tried all sorts of other things on his own. He filled up a bottle of water with actual physical copper, allowed it to sit for hours, removed it, and tested the water: 0 copper. A non-physical copper source (i.e., the energy frequency of copper) created physical copper.

Anything that changes the harmonic frequency is working at the level of energy. Changing the energy changed the physiology of the water—and it changes your physiology, too.

About fifteen years ago I bought my wife, Hope, a dozen roses because I love her so much—and because I wanted to do this experiment. I gave her ten roses, and I took the two that were the most alike of the twelve.

According to the florist, they were grown by the same grower and picked on the same day. My son, Harry, took these pictures and supervised this experiment to make sure it was all done correctly.

I trimmed the roses' stems and put them in a glass of clean water. I took one glass in my hand and very, very intensely remembered the worst, most painful memory of my life. I really tried to put myself back there again, experiencing it all over again. I did that for sixty seconds. Then I put the glass down and never touched it again. Harry made sure of that.

I took the other glass in my hand and very intensely thought about the happiest, best, most loving memory of my life. I tried to relive it all over again for sixty seconds. I put the glass down and never touched it again. After forty-nine hours, here was the result:

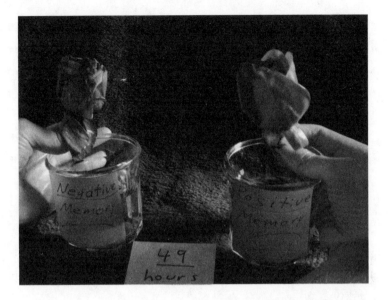

And seven days later:

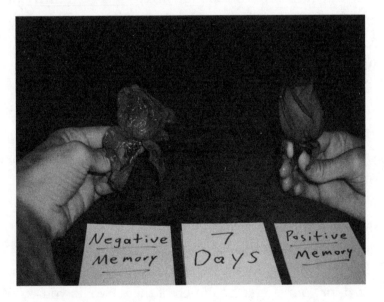

The first time I presented these pictures, someone shouted out from the audience, "It looks like that one has cancer." It had big, black blotches all over it. If you touched it, it was actually slimy. I've never seen a rose get slimy like that. If you took the other one out of the water, the water would run off and it would become perfectly dry.

Hope put the ten roses I gave her in a vase with flower food that makes them last longer. The rose on the right looked better than any of the ten with flower food. The sixty seconds of remembering the positive memory literally had a healing effect on it and kept it from aging as quickly.

This experiment is not original with me. I got it from someone who did it with strawberries. Last year, someone who attended my workshop in Tokyo had read my book and did it at home with white rice. They brought the results to the workshop: one bowl was still completely white. The other one was dark gray with black blotches through it.

This profound difference happened after just sixty *seconds* of negative thinking! Can you remember any day in your life that you did not, for at least sixty seconds, think of something negative? For most people, the answer is no. Personally, I've never had a day where I didn't think of something negative for at least sixty seconds.

Here's the second, and more important, point. Which of these two results do you want to be your liver, your brain, or your stomach? Which of these two do you want to be your children, your career, or your most important relationship?

It's not surprising that we get sick. What's surprising is that we don't get sick more often with all the negative thoughts and feelings going through us. Our immune and healing systems do a miraculous job keeping us as healthy as they do, with the devolution of memory we're all dealing with.

ENERGY MEDICINE FOR MEMORIES: MEMORY ENGINEERING

As we learned in part 1, our memories are the source of our life experiences: thoughts, feelings, physiology, behavior—everything. You are making new memories constantly and instantly, but they are filtered through and built on your existing memories of that same or similar experience. Changing your memories may be the only way you can truly change your life at the source for the better and sustain it long-term.

So how do we change our memories? If everything is energy, our memories are also made of energy. That means we need a solution that can change energy at the source of the problem. You don't use a lug wrench to brush your teeth. You don't use a toothbrush to change your tire. You use the right tool for the right job. And if you've got an energy problem, you need an energy-based solution. We need an energy-based memory changing tool kit or machine. Remember, they have cut out every part of the brain and the memories are still there. They are not flesh and bone, blood or tissue—they are made of energy, just like your computer's hard drive files, text messages, radio, and wi-fi. In fact, computers were designed to work the way *we* work.

Memory engineering is a specific energy medicine/psychology technique that targets our source memories. And that brings us to the next chapter.

CHAPTER EIGHT

Memory Engineering: You Have to See It to Believe It

Memory engineering sounds like something out of a scary science-fiction novel. What in the world do I mean by "memory engineering"?

THE HISTORY OF HEALING MEMORIES IN PSYCHOLOGY

The concept of memory engineering may be brand-new, but the idea of using memories to heal the human condition is not. In fact, it's how psychology began. When Freud—the father of modern psychology—saw his patients, he asked them to lie on a couch, close their eyes, and recount their memories for hours at a time. "Tell me about your mother. Tell me how you felt about that." It was called analysis, and it would typically last for years.

As best I can tell from studying this practice in my doctoral program and knowing colleagues who practice it today (which is unusual), the successful conclusion of analysis is basically when the patient has nothing else to say. They have said it all: every little urge, every inappropriate thought and feeling, everything that happened, everything that didn't happen. They've talked through the memories of their entire life to exhaustion.

If the person had never really talked about what was bothering them before, then it makes sense that they would feel better after talking about it. They were able to share their deepest secrets, thoughts, and feelings with a sympathetic, caring person, and the pressure was relieved. But they're still left with the same memories and may even still feel the same way about most of them. If they rated a memory as a negative 9 in terms of how much it bothered them, perhaps it's now only a negative 3. That is simply a form of desensitization.

Desensitization is not healing; it's like having a smaller wound, but the wound is still there and often still infected, which means it will likely get worse again later. Plus, in the field of psychology, we now know that just talking endlessly about your troubles often makes them worse, not better, even if you are desensitized to them to some degree.

Over time, psychology shifted away from talking to the point of exhaustion because psychologists realized it didn't often change the problem long-term and was very time-consuming and expensive. People felt better, but often only temporarily and partially.

Today, psychology uses three main tools: drugs, coping mechanisms, and more practical approaches like cognitive behavioral therapy and life coaching. Talking about changing your thoughts, emotions, and beliefs has become very popular, and life coaching has taken off like a rocket, because it's a little more practical and positive than just sitting there talking about your mother.

Now, I do believe there is a type of counseling that is very effective, and that is educational or skills-based counseling.

For example, in the early years of our marriage, riding in the car together caused a lot of arguments between Hope and me, because she's an extremely cautious driver (I'd say overly cautious), and I am not the least bit cautious. When I drove, which was almost all the time, I'd go too fast and run up pretty quickly behind somebody; every time she would start mashing her feet on the floor like she had an invisible brake pedal down there, pushing on the dashboard, and even yelling, "Alex!"

I didn't understand it because I had never had a wreck in my life. I still haven't to this day. But then I learned a really simple fact. Men and women have different depth perceptions. Women see things as if they're closer and coming up more quickly than men do.

After I learned that one little thing, driving with Hope was never a problem again. I understood why Hope reacted the way she did. That type of counseling, in which you receive education about the way life works and practical instructions, can work really well.

I would say that easily over 90 percent of what we call "success" in psychology, medicine, and now life coaching is not really a resolution of the problem. It's a significant relieving of pressure—significant enough that the person says, "I feel a lot better." That's how counseling and therapy started, and these are still the threads that run through it today.

The great majority of what people call healing today consists simply of coping and instructions. For that 3 percent of people I mentioned earlier who are going to be successful no matter what, instructions are all they need. For the rest of us, we need extra help understanding the instructions or actually doing them. That leaves us with coping, which either stops working eventually or takes an enormous amount of your daily energy for the rest of your life.

Why does coping take so much energy? Because talking about and reasoning through your problems is primarily a conscious undertaking. At best, you're only dealing with the symptoms. The *source* of the problem is virtually always in the unconscious or subconscious (Dr. Lipton says more than 90 percent of the time) and is actively being protected from being healed because it's labeled as a life-or-death issue. Add to that the fact that your unconscious is more than a million times more powerful than your conscious mind, and hopefully you get the picture. Your conscious says, "That's not a big deal; change it," and your unconscious says, "Thanks for asking, but *no way*."

The result is that most people tend to settle for "okay" in their lives. They settle for 278 problems that are "a lot better"—rather than complete, long-term healing and few if any significant problems.

We tend to be okay with this because of what we said in part 1: we compare ourselves with other people. Let's say you're on three medications, and you're not sure how you feel about that. You talk to one friend about it and discover he's actually on four medications. Then you talk to another friend who tells you she can't find any medication to solve her problem and has trouble getting out of bed each morning.

You say to yourself, *Wow, I feel a lot better about the three medications I'm taking. At least I can get out of bed in the morning. I'm doing fine!*

No, you're not! Quit comparing yourself to other people. You are built for greatness, not just for coping or getting through the day.

I quoted Freud in chapter 1 as saying, "Idealism is the cause of all human suffering." Remember, idealism is *comparison* and *expectation* put together.

Usually we think of idealism as causing suffering when we expect *more* than what we have. But it can cause just as much suffering if you expect *less* than what you *could* have.

Let's not mistake coping for healing anymore. Let's not just desensitize ourselves to our problems. Let's heal the source. Let's go into your memories and change them to produce the kind of positive internal environment you were designed to live in.

MEMORY ENGINEERING RESEARCH

Our memories impact our energy, and that coding lives in our physical bodies. I came to really understand that fully when I heard accounts of organ transplant recipients. Many organ transplant recipients have stated they experience the food cravings and personality characteristics of the donor. One recipient reported a new love for classical music, another reported vivid memories of her donor's murder that led to a conviction, and still another experienced a change in sexual orientation. Most studies hypothesize something in the tissue carries the information of the donor's memories to the recipient, although the evidence is still anecdotal.[1]

Also, according to anecdotal evidence, near-death experiences create very powerful memories that seem to become the new positive default for that individual.

This powerful positive experience seems to "reset" any fear memories and negative internal programming in a way that seems permanent and effortless on the part of the individual.[2] Much like my transformational *aha* after Hope kicked me out of the house.

To me, both of these phenomena are further indication of both the power of our memories and the potential to change them.

Of course, the question is how. We don't just want to hope for a near-death experience or an organ transplant! Psychology has always known that the real source of our problems is in our memories. It just couldn't find a way to fix them consistently and for the long term.

The good news is that it *is* actually possible to change them, and science is beginning to demonstrate this as well.

In the last few decades, researchers have returned to the issue of memories as the source of everything we experience—what psychologists intuitively knew from the beginning. We mentioned several of these studies in part 1. The researchers from Southwestern University said once we figured out how to change our cellular memories, it would be the difference between life and death.[3]

Recently, some researchers have discovered how to change these internal images in ways that measurably change physiology and behavior.

MEMORY ENGINEERING IN MICE

In 2013, MIT neuroscientists discovered that they could make permanent changes in mice's behavior by changing their memories. First, they used genetically engineered mice with two unique characteristics: their neurons would glow red when highly active, and their neurons could be light-activated. This meant the researchers could not only see exactly what neurons were firing in the hippocampus (the area of the brain that creates new memories), but also activate those memories at will by shining light on those neurons.

Here's how they set up the experiment. First, research- ers allowed the mice to explore a new area so they could create a memory of it. Then they removed the mice from that area, shone light on those specific neurons to activate that memory again, and administered electric shocks to make it a fearful one.

When the mice were reintroduced to the original area, they repeatedly exhibited signs of fear they hadn't before. The conclusion was that changing their memories in this way did result in permanent changes in the mice's behav- ior.[4] The title of the *Scientific American* article reporting on this research was "The Era of Memory Engineering Has Arrived."

VIRTUAL REALITY TREATMENT IN HUMANS

That type of memory engineering may work for geneti- cally engineered mice in a lab, but what about humans? Several studies have demonstrated that virtual reality can have similar results with humans—no genetic engineer- ing, lab, or electric shocks required.

In one study, people with Parkinson's disease exer- cised on a treadmill while wearing virtual reality goggles that showed their feet walking on a path in a game. The game allowed them to practice walking normally and avoiding obstacles. Researchers discovered that the virtual reality training increased the neuroplasticity of the participants and improved brain function.[5]

Another study showed that virtual reality can help paraplegics walk again. Researchers initially discovered that when the eight participants in the study were asked to imagine walking, their brains showed no signal at all. According to the lead researcher, Miguel Nicolelis, MD, PhD, of Duke University, "It's almost like the brain had erased the concept of moving by walking."[6] In other words, after their accident, they no longer had any memory or internal image of how to walk.

The researchers used virtual reality, in which participants used brain activity to move an avatar around in a simulation, to essentially give participants a new memory of walking. The participants used this new memory of walking to activate a computerized exoskeleton, and over time, after "walking" in the exoskeleton for an hour a day, all eight participants regained some kind of sensation and/or movement. One woman had been paralyzed for thirteen years, and after the treatment, with her body supported by a harness, she was able to move her legs on her own.[7]

Virtual reality treatment has also helped reduce phantom pain in people with spinal cord injuries.[8] Similar results have been found when using virtual reality treatments on patients with stroke,[9] depression,[10] and pain during hospital stays.[11]

These and other studies have shown that images (i.e., our memories) not only are at the root of every issue in our lives, but also can be altered to create seemingly miraculous and permanent changes downstream.

Now, the skeptics are going to say, "Whoa, wait a minute! Change your memories? You don't want to do that! That's like living a lie."

The truth is, according to what we covered in part 1, you're living the lie right *now*. We want to fix the lie you're living as a result of the memory malfunction. That malfunction is what caused you to live the lie. We want to fix that corrupted file, or human hard drive virus, so your memories are truthful and create love, joy, peace, maximum potential, purpose, and meaning in your life.

HOW I DISCOVERED MEMORY ENGINEERING

Outside the research lab, mainstream medicine, and mainstream psychology, people have been working on healing memories for quite some time. In fact, the practice has been around for centuries or even millennia, primarily in spiritual or religious contexts. I've done it myself in a variety of nonreligious ways: the Healing Codes are a way to heal memories, for example, as is the Heart Screen Meditation from *The Love Code*.

If you are familiar with these practices, you may be wondering, *Is memory engineering different from healing memories? If so, how?*

The quick answer is that it's based on the same principle of energy medicine that those other techniques are based on: we hit the negative frequency of the fear-based memory with a positive frequency, primarily by imagining positive memories to counteract the negative memories, with some very important differences that make it much more effective.

To explain those differences, I need to back up and explain how my quest to help others heal began.

It started in the early years of my marriage, when Hope had been depressed for about six years. She had tried medications and some alternative treatments, and nothing had worked. Her life was still a living hell.

Around that time, I came to believe what I explained in chapter 1: that what Solomon called the heart 3,000 years ago is primarily what psychology calls the unconscious mind, plus some other related things like our right brain and our conscience. It's not quite that simple, but there's a lot of overlap. I found this startling because the Bible and other spiritual manuscripts that talk about the heart say that it's the most important thing in life. It's where all our problems and solutions are found.

I came to believe that Hope's true problem and solution would be found in her heart, which is when my quest shifted to understanding the issues of the heart. What are the issues of the heart? They're lies, or untruths, in our memories. Memories, as we know, are images, and images are the language of the heart.

Earlier I mentioned that because of the devolution of memory, most of our memories have so many errors in them that researchers say they're more like illusions than facts.[12] I also mentioned that for our purposes here every memory can be rated as love-based or fear-based on a scale of negative 10 to positive 10, and your life experience depends on the overall rating of all your memories put together.

For most people, their overall memory ratio is more negative than positive, primarily because of all the errors in their memories. Every error—or lie, you might call it—spikes your stress. The fact that your stress spikes in reaction to a lie is the basic premise behind a lie detector test. It's how we're wired.

What that means for your memories is that every error will push that ratio farther to the negative end of the spectrum. Your negative ratio can also come from the words you think, feel, and use, such as "This weather's killing me," your negative ancestral memories, and all the other issues that contribute to the devolution of memory we discussed in chapter 3.

That's why so many people end up with an overall memory ratio of something like negative 5, and why they wake up each morning feeling like the best they can do each day is barely survive.

If you want to live the best life for you, and truly heal all the problems you know you have, you've got to do something to get that unconscious negative ratio at least into the neutral area, if not the positive. You have to. There's no other way. That's what I mean by healing your issue at the source.

While Hope was depressed, I read every book I could find, and when the Internet became available, I looked up every resource on the Internet. There were all kinds of suggestions for healing memories, but we tried them, and none of them did it for her.

A few years later the study from Southwestern on cellular memory came out, along with the many stories about organ transplant recipients I cited earlier, which showed that memories aren't all located in our brain. So if you have a memory that's causing you to think and feel negative things, get sick, and live a life you don't want to live, is there any way to change it?

I tried all sorts of things myself, and the best program I developed for that purpose was a technique I called reverse hypnosis. It uses guided imagery to take people through every year of their life, and I've seen really wonderful results from it. The problem is that it works best if someone else leads you through it, it takes a long time, and even then it doesn't always work the way you want it to.

During my psychology doctoral program, a few friends and I were fascinated with the idea of healing or changing memories, and we tried various methods and techniques. One of the absurd things we tried was literally screaming at the person the opposite of the troubling problem, using a positive trauma to offset a negative trauma. As you probably guess, it didn't have the desired effect. I may have tried and tested a hundred other things after that, with sometimes better but still disappointing results.

I was still missing something. As it turns out, I was missing three things. We've discussed each of these three issues before, but here's why they are so important for healing memories long term.

Talk to Your Heart as a Partner in Your Healing

I've mentioned before that our heart responds to every activated image in our mind as if it's real and happening right now, and that triggering a negative memory spikes our stress just like the original event.

I also eventually realized that because a lie also spikes our stress, if we're trying to reimagine (or remember) a negative memory in a way that we know is not true, it's going to spike our stress and release even more adrenaline, now making that negative memory more powerful than it was even before the reactivation.

That's why positive affirmations so often don't work in the long term. If you tell yourself, "I'm receiving a million dollars right now," your heart knows you're lying, and your stress spikes every time, creating more of the negative effects you're trying to get rid of. In other words, if I just imagine a positive memory to offset the negative memory, and the positive isn't true, I may have made it worse instead of better! I've tried to fix a lie with another lie, kind of like the old expression "throwing gasoline on the fire."

Here's breakthrough number one. *You have to have a relationship with your heart and include it as a partner in your healing.* Remember, your unconscious is more than a million times more powerful than your willpower, so if they don't work together in harmony, you will always lose. Have regular conversations with your heart. Talk to your heart like a dear friend or relative. What we have to do is join hands with our heart and tell it the truth in love. We can tell it something like, "Thank you so much for helping me do what's best. I'm sorry I've been so hard to deal with. Can we cooperate now? Can we work together to change my negative, erroneous programming to positive, healthy programming?"

In the next chapter, you'll see that the first four (of six) steps in the Memory Engineering Technique give you a chance to join hands and explain to your heart that you know these positive images you're creating are not true; they are for programming reasons only, to neutralize the negative images and errors and create a more positive overall ratio. The last two steps are creating the perfect, truthful, new memories that will become your new default for that issue for the rest of your life.

You don't have to know or change every single negative memory. You only need to create enough positive energy in the mind to neutralize the negative energy and end up with a neutral or positive ratio overall, or related to that particular issue. That's how energy medicine works: you hit a negative frequency with a positive frequency, and it's neutralized or changed to a new positive.

When your heart knows you're not lying to it and working only for your betterment, it comes fully on board with changing your memories, and works with you rather than against you.

Release Your Heart's Safety Features

In part 1, we talked about how your heart's number one job is to keep you physically alive for the first six to twelve years of your life, and it has certain safety features that send in the Fear Response Team whenever you experience anything remotely resembling a fear-based memory. Keeping you physically alive no matter what continues to be its number one priority in adulthood until you discover what all of life is about, choose the Law of Internals, and commit to change in order to live that way. Until then, it has certain safety features turned on. If you can't find a parking place close to the store and start thinking, *I'm going to die if I don't find a parking place soon*, it has no choice but to pull the alarm and send in the Fear Response Team. And all of a sudden, you've gone from a pretty good day to thinking, *What happened to me?*

Our systems are fairly well hardwired. As a safety precaution, the heart will not violate that number one job of self-protection for any reason—*except one*.

You can release your heart's safety features if you choose to live by the Law of Internals: to live in love as best you can in the present moment, regardless of your circumstances or of any end result, from now on—period. This is the meaning and purpose of your life, in my opinion. This can and will work, when you are fully invested in allowing it to work: you have to really mean it and commit to it. You can't fool your heart.

That was my second breakthrough: *To truly heal your issues at the source, you must release your heart's safety features by choosing the Law of Internals*. Otherwise memory healing doesn't last.

Remember, your unconscious knows when you're lying. It knows why you do something when you don't know why you are doing it, and it knows when you do something without being fully committed. You can say it a thousand times, but if you're not really dedicated to it, your heart knows you aren't fully dedicated, and it will keep sending in the Fear Response Team whenever your circumstances trigger your false fear memories created because of the devolution of your memory's meanings.

But the minute you truly commit to love no matter what for the rest of your life, your heart immediately says, "Announcement! We just got it! Release the safety features. Let's fly."

Why? The heart's mandate is to keep you alive until you figure out what life is all about and choose it. If you haven't chosen it yet, the heart will remain guarded. Maybe you'll choose it tomorrow, but until then, you've got to stay alive.

The only thing that's more important than death is love.

As we said in part 1, when and if this ever happens, the heart deprioritizes the fear memories and starts prioritizing the positive love memories. Often the fear memories can even cease to be fearful, as they are changed by the huge new influx of love.

Fear is by definition the absence of love, and it cannot exist in the presence of pure and true love—as opposed to "acting" loving for social acceptance and "what's in it for me."

Turn On Psychological Adaptation

In chapter 1, we talked about psychological adaptation, the mechanism that allows us to adapt to almost any situation, whether they are over-the-moon successes or disastrous tragedies. Psychological adaptation is why, after about six months, lottery winners and paraplegics report the same average level of happiness and satisfaction with their life—versus six months earlier, when it was as different as you can imagine.

Psychological adaptation is largely related to your prefrontal cortex. It is built into every one of us, but here's the problem. When that negative-to-positive ratio gets too negative (my guess is around negative 5 or lower), as I mentioned at the end of part 1, I've found that psychological adaptation doesn't kick in. It tries to, but can't overcome the extreme negativity coming from our fear-based memories. This is why Hope was depressed for twelve years and not just six months. And the same is true for my acid reflux that went on for two or three years. At some point, the negative obstacle becomes too difficult to overcome, and the natural process of psychological adaptation can't kick in without some extra help.

If you could somehow get that ratio down from a negative 7 to a negative 3, psychological adaptation would kick in, and six months from now you'd feel like a different person. *Hey, I'm okay now. I'm really okay. Let's live life!* At negative 7, you may never get to your best life, no matter how many things you try.

Of course, without the devolution of memory, the vast majority of us would never have gotten to negative 7 in the first place. We'd experience difficulties and even tragedies, but psychological adaptation would always kick in eventually and we'd be okay again. But over thousands of years, where now almost anything can trigger the Fear Response Team, many of us are too negative, and we're malfunctioning constantly! And nothing—maybe not even the Healing Codes or any other modality that should be healing the problem at the source—is working enough to offset the trillions of memories interpreted as life-or-death issues throughout your family history. You may get better but never reach your maximum potential.

That was my third breakthrough. *Although it's true that we have the choice to choose love every day, it's almost impossible for us to choose it if our heart environment is too negative.* We're in too much fear. That's what I saw in my clients: they needed to get their heart environment positive enough to be able to choose the Law of Internals.

The Memory Engineering Technique directly addresses all three of those issues that I had been missing over the years. I've tested it out with groups and individuals around the world, and I've never seen anything work as reliably and as quickly for changing negative memories. It first helps your overall heart ratio become more positive so psychological adaptation can kick in, and then it heals both the memory itself and all its related memories to create a new default for that issue, with the right tools for the job.

And you can do memory engineering even if you can't fully commit to the Law of Internals yet. As your heart ratio becomes more positive, you'll become capable of choosing the Law of Internals, enabling your full healing.

THE CONTROL PANEL OF YOUR HEART: YOUR IMAGE MAKER

What are the right tools for the job? Remember, these images aren't made of bone, blood, or tissue. They're made of energy patterns, and that means you need an energy tool to fix them. Memory engineering may sound like something from *Star Trek*, but it's simply an energy-based tool that creates, heals, edits, and revises those images. It's the right tool for the job.

You don't need surgery, drugs, or even an expert practitioner to do it for you. That's because we are already equipped with the internal technology to change our memories: our imagination, or what I call our image maker.

I find it fascinating that medical science cannot find exactly where memories are stored. They have cut out every part of the brain, and the memories are still there. Individuals who have been declared dead and then come back to life are not only able to recall their experiences while "dead," but typically remember these experiences with much more clarity and detail than memories created while they were alive.

We view memories on the screen of our image maker. Science cannot find that screen anywhere. I believe the reason for both of these oddities is that your unconscious memories and the screen you view them on are actually more in the spiritual realm of your internal being. And again, we have no tools to measure that. Why don't critics say your memories or your image maker doesn't exist, as they often do for anything without empirical evidence? Because their existence is so obvious it would make them look ridiculous.

Personally, I believe the image maker is connected to the following physical mechanisms:

The right brain. The language of your right brain is images, and its worldview is spatial rather than linear. It's the source of "out of the box" thinking.

The brainstem. The brainstem is your "feeling brain," which accesses unconscious and generational memories, and their relevant life information, at 286,000 miles per second.

The hippocampus. Its function includes the editing, storing, and recalling of memories.

The amygdala. The amygdala is the seat of emotions and feelings, and the wisdom behind them.

The reticular formation. This part of the brain activates action based on input from all of the elements listed above.

The bottom line is that your image maker generates images, wisdom, wise judgment, out-of-the-box problem solving, peak performance, appropriate action, and enormous power. On the other hand, words are, for all practical purposes, just connected to words.

Your image maker is not a gimmick, and it's not pretend—it's the control panel of your life. It's your direct access to your memories. Memory engineering allows you to sit in the control chair of your heart and heal your images—and therefore all the issues of your life—at the source. You probably never knew that you could monitor and control the images that drive your thoughts, emotions, and behavior. I'm here to tell you that you can. In fact, you must if you want to make the most of the gift of life you've been given.

It's your choice: will you use your image maker to create unreal fantasies and let your real life run on autopilot—seeking pleasure and avoiding pain throughout your whole life? Or are you going to take control and use it to create a new, positive reality for you and everyone around you?

Don't worry; you don't have to be a "visual" person to master the art of memory engineering. As for myself, I have what I can only describe as negative art skills. Whenever my family and friends get together to play games, the one I dread most is Pictionary. Every time I draw my picture, everyone laughs—in both groups. (It doesn't help that my wife, Hope, is an artist.) Sometimes the whole game stops so that someone can say what everyone is thinking: "What in the heck is that?" When I tell them what it is, they are incredulous. "You've got to be kidding! That's the best you could do for that?" It is usually the biggest laugh of the night and gets brought up frequently at later occasions.

The visuals I'm talking about aren't the ones that you create with your hands and the right assortment of crafts. The truth is, everyone is a visual person; they just don't live like they are. Our worldview, our plans, our hopes, dreams, and fears—all of these are structured around visuals that we hold in our minds of how the world is and what we want it to be like. When there's friction, we go around trying to fix things in other ways, thinking that the problem is money, or health, or that someone else isn't doing what we want them to do—we look for exterior solutions to problems that are really rooted in the interior.

The problem is how you're *perceiving* your life through the lens of your internal pictures. Your image maker is how you see and change these internal pictures.

How do these pictures work? Usually we think of pictures as printed on paper—still, permanent, and dead. But our memory images are more like a movie and are alive. They spread and multiply. This means we can't just ignore or lock away our negative memories, and we can't appease them with love substitutes or escape mechanisms or addictions. Not only will "just getting through the day" not work long term, but it will also make things worse. We might be distracted temporarily, but unconsciously those negative memories are still present, continuing to spread and infect surrounding memories. Eventually they'll unconsciously trigger our fear response over and over and over again—we won't know why—and our life will start mysteriously malfunctioning in all sorts of ways.

Here's an example. Let's say you were once romantically interested in someone, and you have a memory of that person being mean to you. How does this memory operate in your image maker?

That memory has two parts, and a critical result of the two parts: The first part is the event itself, what that person said to you. The second part is the *context* of the event, which is also part of the memory. If you were standing on carpet, you have the carpet in the memory. If that person was wearing a green shirt or smelled like a certain perfume, you have a green shirt or a smell in the memory, along with everything else that was a part of that event.

What's also part of this context are all the other memories of your life that are somehow related to that memory. Maybe your parents had previously warned you not to get involved with this person. Maybe your father was wearing a green shirt when he yelled at you when you were small or a stern aunt wore the same perfume. All of these are part of the context.

Let's say this memory is causing you to avoid all romantic relationships today, and you came to see me about it. I would ask you, "What did this person actually say or do?" You think about it, and you say, "Well, he told me, 'I'm not interested in you in a romantic way right now.'"

Wait a minute. *Was* that person mean to you? If I went to that person and asked him about you, maybe he would say, "Oh, I thought the world of her. But you know what? I just had a really bad breakup with someone else and knew I wasn't any good for anybody right then."

Many times, what's really bothering us about a memory is not actually in the event, it's in the context. That context might be something that happened with your parents, or even ten generations ago! The context caused your heart to interpret an event as traumatic, and its negativity spread like a virus—when someone with a completely different context wouldn't interpret it that way at all.

And that's the critical result: the interpretation. Every belief you have is an interpretation of all memories related to that issue. It's like an *if . . . then* statement: Because _____, therefore _____. And we can have conflicting beliefs about the same thing. The one we act on is typically the one that is stronger at the time, and remember, our negative memories tend to be prioritized and are therefore usually the strongest.

What matters is whether the memory is traumatic to *you*. Both the event and the context are real. To truly change the memory, you have to heal both.

If you heal just the event (like the practice of healing memories typically does) and not the context, the negative effects will usually return. If you heal the context without healing the event, the same is true.

Memory engineering heals both the event and the context. We need to change the specific memory, and we need to change the contextual memories—all the memories connected to and surrounding it.

That may sound complicated, but your image maker

does this a thousand times a day. The problem is that we've just let it run on autopilot. Letting your image maker operate on default your whole life is like buying a cell phone and then never setting it up. Six months later, you begin to wonder, *Why can't I text anyone? Why can't I check my email?* So you go to your teenage son and say, "Why doesn't my phone work the way yours does?"

He asks you, "Have you set it up?"

"Well, no."

"Dad, it says you've got a hundred fifty updates here. Have you updated anything?"

"No—I didn't know I needed to do that."

We're walking around with the control panel to our thoughts, feelings, beliefs, behaviors, health, and happiness in our pocket, but all we do is carry it around and keep it charged. We never set it up to work for us. We don't use it to change our thoughts, to change our feelings, to change our beliefs, to change our physiology. We don't even know it will do that.

It's like me saying to my son, "Oh, you mean I can push this button and get email? You mean I can talk to people on the phone? Wow, I didn't know it would do that!"

My son looks at me like I'm an absolute idiot. "How could you possibly carry all that advanced technology around and not use it?"

I do not think you're an idiot, but I hope by now you're beginning to see how much advanced technology we are all carrying around that too many of us haven't even begun to use. Well, our image creation and editing equipment is far more advanced than any computer or cell phone. We've got to take control of it, set it up, and use it to do all the positive things it was designed to do, rather than let it default to the negative malfunctions.

Memory engineering is one way you can take over your control panel. In the next chapter, you're going to learn exactly how to do that for yourself. But first, let's practice a bit.

PRACTICE USING YOUR IMAGE MAKER

You can practice using your image maker in an unlimited number of ways—you can literally imagine anything you want!

Try this example: Close your eyes and imagine eating a piece of candy. Now imagine the piece of candy explodes into orange juice in your mouth. Play around with that image a few times and note what you see, feel, smell, taste, hear, and experience. You've just used your image creator and your image editor to create a new experience, and then to change it.

Try this next example: Having read this far, can you think of at least one memory that's causing you problems today? Imagine it as an object, imagine watching it on a screen, imagine it however you want but as something that is tangible outside of your own mind. For instance, let's say you struggle with worrying. How would you represent that visually? If you were going to make a movie clip or a picture that represented you worrying, what would it look like to you?

It's possible that nobody on the planet knows about this memory and how it affects you but you. Maybe you're seeing a picture of yourself with a worried expression on your face—your brow is scrunched up and you're gritting your teeth. See whatever comes up for you.

Now, what has to happen in that picture to change the worrying to peace? Change the picture so that you're not worrying and you're at peace. Do it right now. What did you change in that picture? How did that change what you felt?

That's how simple the basic underlying principle of this technology is! You just need to keep doing that from all different angles until you actually feel peace—in real life, not just in your imagination.

Because our heart treats every memory as present-tense reality, any bad experience that happened when we were children didn't just happen twenty years ago; it's happening now in our heart. The good news is that we can quite literally travel back in time to correct that memory from twenty years ago—because it's happening right now. Remember this the next time you are fantasizing or daydreaming, and instead fantasize or daydream intentionally for the positive.

The bottom line is that our memories are alive and powerful. They're organic, they're real—and we can't wish them away. We can't hide from them. If we want to live our best life and not just a life of survival and mediocrity, we must learn to understand our memory images and fix the ones that are lying to us. And the only thing that changes an internal picture is not surgery, not drugs, but another picture. In the next two chapters, you will learn how to do that for yourself using the Memory Engineering Technique.

CHAPTER NINE

The Memory Engineering Technique: Travel Back in Time to Change Your Present and Future

The Memory Engineering Technique is a form of energy medicine that heals both the event and context of your memories by creating positive and/or truthful images to neutralize the negative images, which in turn creates positive, permanent changes in all thoughts, feelings, beliefs, physiology, and behaviors related to that memory. Then you can easily change the conscious interpretations of your day-to-day events.

In addition to most memory or imagery-based healing practices, memory engineering includes three specific breakthroughs:

1. Telling the truth to your heart and fully involving it as a positive partner in your healing.
2. Healing the overall environment of your heart so that psychological adaptation can kick in.

3. Releasing your heart's safety features by choosing the Law of Internals.

The goal of the Memory Engineering Technique is to shift your overall negative heart ratio to neutral or positive, one issue at a time.

Are you ready to start changing your own memories so they create the most positive life for you? Then let's get to work.

THE MEMORY ENGINEERING TECHNIQUE WORKSHEET

First of all, I invite you to go to mymemorycode.com and print out the Memory Engineering Technique worksheet. This worksheet has two parts: on the front is a fill-in-the-blank chart, and on the back is the heading "My Story,"

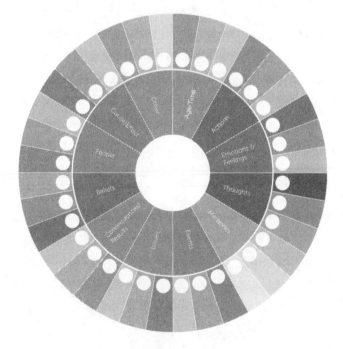

where you can write out the story of your experience in a more open-ended way. You can use either one of these approaches or both.

You do not have to use this worksheet if you don't want to. Hope would fill out one of these every time she used the technique and stress over whether she did it all exactly right. I never fill one out at all. You do what supports you best. I would recommend trying to fill it out at least once so you can decide. Some have found it helpful to fill it out the first time, to really see how this issue affected them in many areas of their lives, and then didn't feel the need to fill it out again.

To use the worksheet, begin by filling in the date so you can track your progress. Fill in your name if you'd like, especially if you and your partner are working on issues together and you don't want to get the worksheets mixed up. Write down the issue you're working on. Finally, write down which version of the worksheet it is, which also allows you to track your progress. Is it the first time you've worked on this or the tenth?

Once you've filled in the top part, you can move to the circle.

Issue

Our goal with memory engineering is to create new memories that start to move our overall heart ratio from negative to positive, and then change the default memory from fear/falsehood to love/truth. We do that with one issue at a time—in this case, I'm going to start with an issue that used to bother me a lot: acid reflux. I might have other issues, like my marriage or my job, which I can address separately on a different worksheet. It's best to start with the issue that's bothering you the most.

Here I wrote down "acid reflux" in the middle of the circle.

Experiences Related to the Issue

The circle is then divided into different pie pieces that name all the related experiences, including the memories (both events and context) and the symptoms resulting from those memories (thoughts, emotions and feelings, beliefs, and actions). Fill in the blanks around the wheel that are relevant to your experience, and rate each item on a scale from 0 to 10, where 0 means it doesn't bother you at all, and 10 means it is an overwhelmingly negative problem in your life. This allows you to get an overall rating for the issue and track your progress over time.

For example, what emotions and feelings was I experiencing because of my acid reflux? I was afraid I was going to get cancer of the esophagus, so under Emotions & Feelings, I wrote down "fear of cancer," and rated it as a 9. I also wrote down "anger," because it was interfering with my daily life, as a 6.

What people were related to this issue? I put Hope, because it affected Hope and me, at about a 7.

What actions are related to this issue? Acid reflux affected what I ate and drank, so I wrote down "diet," a 5. I was taking medication for it, so I also wrote down "medication," a 3.

For thoughts, which are very close to emotions, I wrote down, "Am I going to get cancer?" at a 7.

Note that you don't have to fill in all of these spaces—just those that are significant to you. Also note that you don't have to use a numerical scale to rate your problem. If you have trouble coming up with a number, just note whether it bothers you or not.

PROGRAMMING MEMORY 1: PAST GENERAL

With the Memory Engineering Technique, we are going to create some new, very powerful positive memories, even though we haven't had anything powerful and positive happen. How do we do that? More important, how do we do that without the unconscious rejecting or labeling it as a lie, which could make the problem worse?

In order for memory engineering to work, we have to do it in cooperation with our heart. Our conscious and unconscious are designed to work together in harmony. How are we going to do that? The same way you would with any relationship—we are going to kindly, lovingly communicate until we have a trusting relationship. You're going to start talking to your heart, your unconscious, your subconscious, your conscience, your Higher Self—whatever you want to call it. If each of these terms mean different things to you, include all of them. I would also highly recommend asking God or your higher power to directly and miraculously intercede as well.

Remember, what the heart ultimately wants is for us to figure out the purpose of our life and choose to fully commit to the Law of Internals and live that way. That's what our very existence is about. My heart (and yours) wants us to get there, and it's willing to help if we work in harmony with it and it knows we're trying.

Let's say my overall heart ratio is a negative 7, and I start talking to my heart, trying to make this work. I say, "Heart, I am going to fully commit to love." Heart says, "Nope. He doesn't mean it. He isn't telling the truth. We are not going to cooperate." But what if I'm at a negative 7 and I say, "Heart, I cannot fully commit yet. I would like to and I'm going to start trying right now, but I know I'm not there yet." Heart says, "*Attention, everybody!* Something is changing. He's telling the truth. All right, let's help him."

It doesn't matter what that truth is. Maybe the truth is, "Heart, I cannot imagine being able to fully commit to love. I don't think I'm ever going to be able to do it. But I would like to. Will you help me try to go in that direction?" What is the heart's reaction? "*Attention!* He's telling the truth. He doesn't think he can get there. Let's help him get there."

Are you getting the idea? It doesn't matter how negative you feel if you can be honest about it. Change starts to really take hold when you acknowledge the distance between where you are and where you want to be, communicate lovingly, and ask for help.

The reason this is so important is because we're going to create some memories, on purpose, that are not factually accurate. Yes, you read that correctly. If we just make them up and imagine they are the truth, that means they'll be identified as lies, and it won't work. The heart won't buy it. "Nope, that's a lie. Spike the stress. Pull the alarm. No lies!"

Here's what makes the difference. *We're telling the truth about it.* I'm not presenting it to the heart as being true. In fact, I'm going to request of my heart that it *never* label this memory as being true, but that it accept the memory for positive programming purposes only (to help offset the erroneous negative programming I've inherited and contributed to what's already there).

I've got millions of memories I don't even know I have, going back hundreds of years. Based on the latest research, almost every memory I have has errors or lies in it. That's what is causing a great deal of my problems. The ones we're going to create are not lies, because we're not presenting them as true. A lie is defined as "an attempt to deceive." We are doing the opposite of that. We are acknowledging this is not the truth of what happened, and it's not presented as the truth of what happened. We're asking the heart to only use these images for one purpose: as positive energy to move the overall negative energy ratio a little bit more toward the positive side. Each of these memories we will be creating will essentially be like an antivirus software program you load onto your computer. It has nothing to do with changing what your computer is supposed to do. Its purpose is only to stop the malfunction so the computer can work the way it's designed to work.

When you present it that way, in cooperation with the heart, the heart will not pull the alarm. It won't label it as the truth, but it will shift that energy a little more toward the positive.

In the Memory Engineering Technique, we are going

to create four new memories that are not true, for programming purposes only, and two that are true. We're going to ask that the two new true ones become the new default memories for that issue, forever. We know, because of the negative experiences we're having, that the current default memory is full of lies. For years, I tried to make this technique work with just the two new true memories. It worked for some people, but most people's heart environments were too negative for that alone to do it. They needed more power, more positive energy, to hit that threshold so that psychological adaptation could kick in. I also tried to make it work by asking people to just imagine that the positive happened instead of the negative. That made things worse, because it was interpreted as a lie.

That's what the first four programming memories are for. They allow you to develop a truthful, trusting relationship with your heart and shift your overall heart ratio to the threshold it needs to allow psychological adaptation to kick in, so you can truly heal.

I'm going to use my acid reflux to demonstrate. I've rated it at a 9. I've identified the emotions, feelings, thoughts, and everything else I thought was relevant. I begin with a prayer asking God that the actual problem (in my case, the acid reflux) be miraculously healed, and that the underlying memories be created, edited, and changed however is best.

Now I'm ready to talk to my heart. I'm going to get comfortable, take slow, deep breaths from my stomach, and close my eyes. I say something like this:

Dear Heart, thank you so much for loving and caring for me. Thank you for protecting me when I'm not strong enough to protect myself.

Thank you for always having my best interest at heart. I'm sorry I've made your job so much harder over the years.

Will you please let me join hands with you? Can we please work together in harmony?

I would love to commit to the Law of Internals and live a life of love. I also know if I say that I am committed to that right now, I will not be telling the truth. It may take a long time, but I want to start taking baby steps in that direction. I know I'm not strong enough to do it because I've tried many times and failed. Will you please help me? Will you please help move my energy from negative to positive? Neutralize the thousands of lies in my heart, some that I know about and some that I don't. You know all of them.

Will you please help me shift the energy about acid reflux and whatever is related to it? Please activate all internal healing mechanisms and my internal intelligent healer to heal the physical, spiritual, and mental issues related to this acid reflux. And God, I ask you to please miraculously intervene and heal everything related to this issue. My fear about cancer related to the acid reflux, how that's affected my relationship with Hope, my job, my joy and peace, my anger over having to deal with this—please help me shift these things to positive.

I want to create a new memory for programming purposes only. Do not ever label it as the truth, because you know and I know that it is not the truth. Please make it super powerful to neutralize the lies and the negative energy about these same things. Please accept it as positive programming to help with my negative programming, but never label it as the truth. Please do not spike my stress, because I'm being honest and truthful about this and it is only for those programming purposes.

These are not magic words. It's just what comes up from my heart and my experience doing this with others. You say what comes up from your heart with the same intention expressed above.

Now, I'm going to relax and imagine, which is another way of saying "create a new memory." I'm going to create a new positive memory that what has happened with my acid reflux is not what really happened, and that what really happened was positive, not negative.

Go with whatever comes up in your mind and heart. For me, I'm imagining that I never got acid reflux in the first place. I have no fear of cancer, no discomfort when eating, no anger, no anxiety, and no problem in my relationship with Hope. It never happened. Instead, I spend all that time experiencing living in the moment, doing work I enjoy, having fun, spending time with my family, and relaxing.

I'm going to immerse myself in that memory—taste it, touch it, smell it—until I feel it. If you can't visualize it, no problem; just say the words that describe it in detail. The more you feel it, the more powerful the memory, and the greater positive movement in that issue and your overall heart energy.

For me, right now as I'm actually doing this, I feel joy and happiness. *Ha ha! No acid reflux. Never happened.* That's what I was waiting for. Then I say to my heart, *Thank you, Heart, for helping me. Please make that memory more and more powerful to offset the negative energy about everything related to this and similar things for the rest of my life.*

PROGRAMMING MEMORY 2: PAST MIRACULOUS

Now, I'm going to create a second new memory. This one will also be in the past, but it will not just be positive, it will be a miraculous, unbelievable, once-in-a-lifetime event related to the issue.

First, I say to my heart, *Heart, please never label this memory*

as being true, either, because it is not. Accept and label it for program-
ming purposes only. Make it super powerful to offset the lies and negative
energy in my heart for the rest of my life.

In my second memory, it's not just that I never got
acid reflux, but I go see my doctor for a checkup, and
he says, "Alex, you're the healthiest guy for your age that
I've ever seen in my life. Your physical, your blood work,
your CT scan, everything! Good night, I've never seen
results like this!" He calls the nurse in and says, "Look
at this guy!" He goes to another doctor and says, "You
won't believe this one patient I have. He's twenty-eight
years old, but look, it's like his biological age and health is
twelve. This guy will probably live to be over a hundred."

I keep imagining this event until I feel it. This feeling
should be something like, "Wow! This is like winning
the lottery! I guess I don't have to worry about my health
anymore, maybe ever!"

PROGRAMMING MEMORY 3: PRESENT MIRACULOUS

For the third memory, we're going to create a memory
of what life would be like today if that past miraculous
event actually happened.

I might begin by saying to my heart, *Okay, Heart,*
thank you for your help with that. This next memory about the present
time, please accept this for programming purposes only. Never label this
as the truth because it's not the truth, and I know it is not the truth.
Please make it more and more powerful over time to offset the negative
erroneous memories related to this issue and my heart in general.

What I imagine for this memory is myself right here,
right now, in the present moment, remembering when that

miraculous thing happened in the past. How do I feel right now in the present when I remember that miraculous thing happening? I see it until I feel it. For me, that feeling is joy and relief: "Wow! That was awesome. I guess I don't have to worry about my health anymore. That's fantastic!" I can eat at the spicy barbecue rib place I love, and I don't have to worry about bringing my medicine or being embarrassed when I have to take it in front of my friends. In fact, I can eat whatever I want. My fear of having cancer of the esophagus, which I thought about fifty times a day, is gone. In its place are love, joy, peace, enjoying my work, and enjoying each moment.

Thank you, Heart, for helping me with that.

Just like the virtual reality treatment gave paraplegics a new picture of how to walk, we're giving you a new positive picture for this issue in your life.

PROGRAMMING MEMORY 4: FUTURE MIRACULOUS

For the final programming memory, we're going to imagine what the future will be like if those past and present miraculous memories happen. It could be a year from now, twenty years from now, or at the end of your life. You can choose one of these options, or you could create several memories at different times in the future.

I begin again by saying to my heart, *Heart, please accept this for programming purposes only. Never label it as the truth because it's not. I know it's not. I'm not presenting it as the truth. Please magnify it and make it more and more powerful over time.*

For me, as I imagine it right now, I'm picturing the end of my life, remembering all those wonderful years of fabulous health. The feeling I have is deep relief and joy, almost beyond words. *I truly haven't had the health problems that everyone else I know has had—wow, what a blessing!*

I imagine that until I feel it. The more you can feel it, the better!

Thank you, Heart, for helping me with that.

DEFAULT MEMORY 1: NEW DEFAULT

This next memory will be our first new default memory, where the original event still happened, but we change our negative, erroneous interpretation to a positive, truthful one.

I begin by saying to my heart, *Heart, please help me create this next memory. Make it wonderful and perfect, and please accept this memory for the rest of my life as the truth about this issue. Anytime something happens in my life that might be related to this memory, please activate this memory as the default memory for this issue powerfully and forever. Also activate the first four memories I created to offset any unconscious negative memories, so that this memory can freely act as the default for this issue for the rest of my life. And let me consciously support that by focusing only on this truth related to this issue.*

The memory I create for my first default memory is what actually happened, so in my memory, I still have acid reflux. What is different about this memory compared to my original negative default memory is that this one does not have the lie in it.

Remember, I said the problem was never the event, it was the wrong interpretation we give to the event. I was believing lies about my acid reflux. I wasn't anywhere close to getting cancer of the esophagus, but I had gotten the idea that I was, and it had grabbed hold of me.

I remember the morning I had my follow-up doctor's appointment at Vanderbilt Hospital in Nashville. Before I went, I found Hope, hugged her, and said, "I love you so much," kind of like I was saying goodbye to her and I wasn't coming back. I had this wonderful, spiritual book that meant a lot to me, and I said, "Honey, if anything happens to me [I didn't want to scare her too much], make sure Harry reads this book when he gets older." I truly believed I was about to die! It was never true, but it became true to me. The doctor told me an hour later, when he was looking at my throat, "Oh, no, you don't have any problems that are serious." But I believed I did before he said that.

The new, truthful, default memory is the true event but without the lies of the negative, wrong interpretation. Yes, I have acid reflux, but I'm taking steps to heal it. It's nothing serious I need to worry about in the present or the future. There are only life lessons to learn from it that will make me a better person.

Here's another way you can identify the lie in your memory. Do you have any "because/therefore" beliefs about this memory? "Because I have acid reflux, therefore I'm going to get cancer and die." "The budget is tight this month, therefore I am going to lose the house and not be able to feed the family." "Because I was raped, therefore I'm a piece of meat, I'm dirty, nobody will ever look at me, I'm never safe." What is that belief for you?

The problem is not the "because." The "because" is true. I do have acid reflux. The budget might be tight. People do get raped. The lie, though, is always in the "therefore."

So the new default memory is the actual truth we know, along with the most positive thoughts and feelings about that issue that are possible. Instead of "I've got acid reflux, and I'm going to get cancer and die," the interpretation becomes, "I've got acid reflux, but that does not mean anything negative about the rest of my life. I can have a great life. The acid reflux can go away. I can still be happy, healthy, and successful." That is also the truth.

I'm not saying that is what is going to happen. Only God knows that. I'm saying that as far as I know, it *can* happen. It's my hope, prayer, and desire. I can still be successful, happy, and healthy in my life even though I have acid reflux today. In other words, you combine the most positive possible "therefore" infused with positivity and hope.

I create that memory with that new, truthful interpretation until I feel it. The more I feel it, the better. *Yes, I've got acid reflux, but I can still be happy, healthy, and successful, and it can go away.*

After creating that memory, I say, *Thank you, Heart, for your help with that. Please make this memory super powerful and the default memory for this issue for the rest of my life. It is not for programming purposes. It is to be labeled as the truth.*

DEFAULT MEMORY 2: ULTIMATE DEFAULT

Finally, we create our sixth memory, our second and ultimate default memory. Here we give our heart full permission to create the best possible default memory for us about this issue, based on everything it knows about us and what is in our subconscious and unconscious. This includes ancestral memories we do not know and can't access and any other related issues we may not connect to this issue.

Okay, Heart, memory number six. I want to thank you so much for your help with this. I hope I'm doing this right. I hope what I'm doing is okay with you. Let me know how to change it if it is not okay with you. I know you are a million times more powerful than my conscious mind is. You know everything about me, even things I don't know.

For this sixth memory, please allow me to completely let go of control and for you/spirit/God to create the perfect default memory about this acid reflux issue. If you want me to see it, show it to me. If you don't want me to see it, that's fine, too. I trust you. Please create the perfect, most powerful memory that neutralizes all the negative about this issue forever. Help me to keep taking steps toward committing completely to a life of love. Please label this sixth memory as the ultimate default memory for this issue for the rest of my life. Please change it whenever and however it needs to change.

Relax. Give up control of your imagination. If you see something, great. If you don't, that's fine. Stay there until you feel something. The more you feel it, the better.

As you allow your heart to take control of the healing process, you may begin to remember something that happened to a family member in a previous generation that you believe may be related to the issue you're experiencing. If so, you can use the Memory Engineering Technique on that particular memory as well to get at the issue from an even deeper level.

However, in my experience, people less often see their ancestral memories play out in their mind like a movie (although this has happened) and more often see a picture or metaphor that results in the same emotion that the original event created.

The heart loves to use metaphors. For example, as you're allowing your heart to create its own default memory, let's say you see a really messy, gooey mud puddle. Or maybe you have the feeling you would get if you looked at a messy mud puddle.

Don't think, *This is stupid! Why in the world am I thinking of a mud puddle? I'm making this up. This isn't working.*

Instead, say thank you! Ask your heart, *Whatever this mud puddle represents, please heal it at the deepest level.*

The great spiritual teachers often taught with parables rather than complex concepts. The heart does the same thing. Instead of seeing a movie about how one of your ancestors lost his mother when he was five, or felt completely blocked in his career, or felt ashamed when her father was sent to prison, you might see a run-down, empty house, a big rock, or a mud puddle.

If a therapist was working with a four-year-old whose close family member had just died, the therapist wouldn't talk to them about the concept of death; the child wouldn't understand that. Instead, the therapist might use a metaphor about how the child may be feeling or have the child draw a picture.

In this case, we're the four-year-old, and our heart is the one trying to help us. It may give you a metaphor that is exactly right for healing your issue. You don't need to know the original event, and you don't even need to know what the metaphor means. You can just allow your heart to do what it knows to do at the unconscious level.

After creating all six memories, rate how much your issue is bothering you again on a scale of 0 to 10, or if you'd rather not use a numerical scale, just note whether it bothers you or not.

Let's say my acid reflux issue moved from a nine to a five. That's great, but I also know that's still not far enough. That's okay. You can repeat this process as many times as you need to until the issue no longer bothers you. That's why the worksheet has a place for you to write down the version. I may have to create thirty different memories about my acid reflux before the overall issue shifts to neutral. But every step is an important one, and slowly you will begin to feel the difference. Just talk to your heart the same way every time, and imagine it until you feel it.

If you do repeat the process, the truthful default memory doesn't have to change, unless you realize at some point that there's another positive angle you hadn't thought of before.

It can also change if something negative happens—but here's how. Let's say I go back to the throat doctor in six months and he says, "Alex, I'm sorry to tell you that you have cancer of the esophagus." That's new information that changes the truth of my situation. But instead of adding "I'm going to die of cancer of the esophagus" to my programming memory, I can add "cancer of the esophagus" to the default memory and still have a positive "therefore." For example, "I've got cancer of the esophagus, but that can absolutely heal. As far as I know I can still have a great, successful, wonderful, healthy life." Including a positive message is critically important to the healing process. It's about the positive/negative memory ratio in your heart. If the ratio is too negative, psychological adaptation won't work, and your body and mind won't be able to return to their natural positive default and heal what needs to be healed.

The ultimate default memory that your heart creates can change at any time. Every time you create a new memory for programming purposes only, you can also say, *Heart, if you would like to revise your ultimate default memory on the basis of this new esophagus cancer, please do that.*

USING THE MEMORY ENGINEERING TECHNIQUE

Now you try it. If you'd like to see a video demonstration of the Memory Engineering Technique, go to mymemorycode.com.

1. Use the chart or don't use the chart. Pick an issue and rate it from 0 to 10. The issue could be physical or non-physical. It could be your relationship with a person. I would recommend choosing whatever is bothering you the most.
2. Get comfortable, take some deep breaths from your stomach, and close your eyes if that helps you focus. Say a prayer about the issue and its healing: *God, I ask you to please miraculously intervene and heal everything related to [name the issue]. Please allow my immune system, intelligent healing systems, and this memory engineering process to work at 100 percent efficiency and power.*
3. Then address your heart. If you are doing this at home, I recommend talking out loud to your heart, but you don't have to if that's

uncomfortable. You can say something like, *Heart, thank you for taking care of me, for loving me, for always having my best interest at heart. I'm sorry if I'm stubborn at times. I'm sorry for being too fear-based a lot of the time. I want to live a life more of love if I can do that. Please help me do that. Please help me create these memories so that they will help and not harm me. Please accept this first memory for programming purposes only. It is not true, and I'm not presenting it as being true. Use it only to shift my negative heart ratio from negative to positive.*

Now, create your new imagined memory of the past, substituting the real, negative experience with a positive one. Imagine that. Taste it, touch it, smell it, and stay immersed. Continue until you feel a shift to the positive thoughts, feelings, emotions, and possibly even physical sensations you might feel if it was actually happening in your life.

4. *Heart, please accept this next memory for programming purposes only. It is not the truth, and I do not present it as the truth. Use it only to shift negative energy to positive.* Now, imagine that the negative issue is not what happened, but what happened is the miraculous thing, the fabulous thing, the incredible thing, the once-in-a-lifetime positive thing—again, until you feel that shift.

5. *Heart, please accept this next memory for programming purposes only. It is not the truth, and I do not present it as being the truth. Use it only to shift negative energy to positive.* Imagine that you are exactly where

you are, in the present moment, and you are remembering that wonderful, miraculous reality. How does that make you feel in this present moment, as you remember what happened? Imagine that until you feel the shift.

6. *Heart, please accept this next memory for programming purposes only. Never label it as the truth. It is not the truth, and I do not consider it to be the truth. Use it only for shifting negative energy to positive.* Imagine you are sometime in the future, one year later, ten years later, or even at the end of your life. At that age, you are remembering the wonderful, miraculous reality related to this issue. How would you feel at that point in your life if that was what had actually happened? Imagine it until you feel the shift.

7. *Heart, for this next memory, please accept and label it as the truth about this issue. Make it my default memory for this issue for the rest of my life. Any time anything happens in my life related to this issue, please activate the first four created memories to offset my negative programming, and also activate this memory as the truth about this issue.* Imagine the current truth about the issue, but without the negative "therefore," infused with all the positives that can still happen in your life in spite of that issue—again, until you feel the shift.

8. *Heart, please help me to let go of control. Please create the perfect, most powerful default memory for this issue. Let it be the ultimate default memory for this issue whether I ever see it and know what it is or not. Thank you.*

> 9. Rate your issue again, from 0 to 10. Notice
> any change. Open your eyes.

Go through that sequence, and do each step until you feel it. Maybe one memory you feel after one minute, while another takes you five minutes. That's okay. It takes however long it takes.

It may seem like this technique has a lot of steps. However, today I can do all of these steps in about two minutes. The more you practice it, the more you develop a trust relationship with your heart, and the faster the healing can happen. At first, my heart just kind of stood back and said, "What in the heck are you doing?" But over time, it began to understand and cooperate, so that what first took a long time now takes just a couple minutes. The same thing happened for my clients, and I believe the same thing will happen for you.

AUTOSTREAMING MEMORY ENGINEERING TECHNIQUE

After you've been practicing the Memory Engineering Technique for a while, you may find you don't need to follow the steps above quite as closely. If so, you may want to try a stream-of-consciousness version called the Autostreaming Memory Engineering Technique, where you supervise rather than control the process. That means you will need to be able to trust your heart enough to let go of control and go with the flow. Even for those who have practiced this technique for a while and are able to internally let go of control, I'd only recommend it if you are very visual. All of us are visual in our unconscious, but not all of us can easily access those images through our conscious mind.

I happen to be a very visual person, so the stream-of-consciousness version works well for me. The intention is to ask our heart to create all six memories, let go, and watch what happens. Instead of telling my heart exactly what to do and when, I'm supervising it. I allow my mind, heart, spirit, and hopefully God to create and edit the six memories however they want to, but I'm also taking notes and making sure all the memories are created.

For example, after I ask my heart to create all six memories, I may see the new past positive memory and the first default memory pretty quickly. Then the process may stop. At that point, I would say to my heart, *I haven't seen the past miraculous memory. Can you show me that one, please?* Then I would allow the process to continue, asking to see any missing memories as needed, until all six have been created (with the possible exception of the miraculous default memory, since we don't always see that memory directly).

I now typically use the Autostreaming version every day. Here is the process I follow:

1. Identify and rate your issue as above.

2. Get comfortable and say a prayer for your healing as above, where you ask God or your higher power to miraculously intervene and heal the issue completely, and allow your immune system, intelligent healing systems, and this memory engineering process to work at 100 percent efficiency and power.

3. Ask your heart to create all six memories in its own order and in its own way: *Heart, for [name the issue], please cre-*

ate a past positive memory, a past miraculous memory, a present miraculous memory, and a future miraculous memory. Please do not accept these memories as the truth, but for positive programming purposes only. And please create my new default memory, without the negative "because/therefore" belief, and my new miraculous default memory. Please treat these two default memories as the truth about this issue whenever I encounter anything similar in my life.

4. Then, I just sit back and watch. If the process stalls, I ask my heart to show me the missing memory, until all six memories have been created. If I ask for the miraculous default memory and don't see that one, I simply trust it has been created and let it go.

5. When all six memories are complete, I rate the issue again, as described above. If the issue is still bothering me, I may repeat the process right then, or I may wait to repeat it later, until the issue no longer bothers me.

If you try this version and are struggling with it, no problem—simply return to the previous version.

FAQ

How often should I use the Memory Engineering Technique, and how long should it take?

I'd immediately start doing this process every day on whatever issue you feel is the worst for you.

If you're a perfectionist, I would strongly encourage you to keep it simple, like the acid reflux example above. Even if you want to use the worksheet, you may find it more helpful to skip it and see what happens. Trust your heart.

Also, sometimes the change is instant, and sometimes it's a process. You may create the new series of six memories and rate the issue at a 3 when you're done. That's terrific, but tomorrow you should go back and check them, to see if they're still strong and intact. If not, repeat the process and put them back on track.

Creating the memories themselves can also be a process. Some people create them in five seconds or less every time, no problem. Those tend to be people who are good at visualizing, who see things pretty easily, or have a good imagination. Actually, everyone has a good imagination; it's just that with some people, the heart has shut down their imagination because it's continued to imagine such negative things that it is hard for the person to get through the day. Sometimes, to protect you, your heart takes your ability to visualize away, but it'll typically come back as you heal.

Maybe one person in thirty needs multiple sessions to create these pictures in the first place. It's extremely rare, but it does happen. If that's you, don't sweat it. Just complete the multiple sessions, and then check your memories every day for about three or four days to make sure they're staying strong and intact. If they've changed, just revisualize them again.

If you've worked on the issue for some time but still notice negative thoughts, beliefs, feelings, and behaviors, you may need to work on some other related memories, too. You have trillions and trillions of memories. For example, if you're worried about your job, that worry may come from 150,000 different memories, not just the two you've been reengineering. Other memories may come from your personal experience, your parents, your friends, other people whom you know, or what you were taught in school, and every time you think about it again or something happens in your life that your mind decides is related to that memory, it's reactivated. Plus, every time it's reactivated it can create a new negative memory or alter the ones you have. That's how our memories are more like illusions than video recordings.

Maybe you reengineer that single memory, which heals 10,000 related memories, and you feel way better for eight hours or a day or longer. But then you start worrying about your job again. You didn't start worrying again because the process didn't work. You started worrying again because you've still got 140,000 memories that aren't healed yet.

The good news is that you never have to address 150,000 memories individually, because they're all in the same file folder. Remember, our memories are linked by our interpretation. They're all connected. When you reengineer one memory with a certain interpretation—such as a memory of getting in trouble as a child for not finishing your work on time, which you interpreted as "when I don't finish my work on time, I'm a bad person"—that single process can reengineer all the memories with that interpretation. I'd recommend working on the earliest and most painful related memories you can, and you'll likely heal a lot at once.

I would say at least 50 percent of people will go through this process once and all the nonphysical symptoms will be gone. Over time this will typically translate to physical symptoms, too.

To make a long story short, be patient. The process takes longer for some people than others, and that's okay.

I am experiencing general anxiety, but I can't identify a specific issue. Can I still use the Memory Engineering Technique?

If you have general anxiety but can't point to a specific memory or issue, I would take the chart and fill it out based on what you're thinking, feeling, and believing right now. On the back of the chart, you can write your story about this. How long has it been going on? How bad is it? Is it worse sometimes than others? If so, what's going on during those times? Is it worse during morning or night? Then, form a picture in your mind based on what you just filled out, and start working on that picture. Do the process on it, and then, if you need to, you can identify your earliest or most painful memory that shares the biggest negative feeling with what you're experiencing right now, and work on that. But very often you don't have to. When you deal with just your unknown issue based on your symptoms, it forms the correct picture that connects to the correct memories in your unconscious and works the same way.

What if I'm not sure the images I'm seeing are coming from my heart? What if I am consciously creating these images?

You can say consciously, "My intention for the next few minutes, as best I can, is to let go of control and let my heart provide the image." You can even say, *Heart, I'm not very good at letting go of control, so I'm going to try to do this, but I don't know if I'll do it very well or not. You're a million times more powerful than me. Even if I can't let go of control, override me and make the image you want—even if I think I did it consciously.*

**Is there anything else I can do to help shift the
thoughts, feelings, beliefs, and other issues
downstream of the memories, besides the Memory
Engineering Technique?**

In addition to the technique itself, keep reminding
yourself that the reason you are having these negative
experiences is not because of your circumstances. Trying
to get more money, or a better job, or even to recover
from a health problem is not necessarily going to move
you farther toward a positive heart ratio, because your
circumstances weren't causing your negative experiences.
The issue is internal, not external. That means your focus
should be internal.

Another simple practice I've seen incredible results
from is this: any time you have a negative thought or feeling, do not allow it as a thought or feeling. Instead, turn it
into a prayer. After every negative thought or feeling you
notice, simply ask, *Please turn this negative thought/feeling into a
positive thought/feeling.* Even if you have to do it a hundred
times a day. Turning it into a prayer instead of just thinking it as a thought changes the energy from negative way
over to positive. It's incredible!

For about three weeks, you'll probably feel like this
practice is driving you insane, because you have to do
it so often. But there will come a time where the heart
shifts. It's almost like the heart says: *Okay, we get it. Any negative thoughts or feelings you're going to turn into a prayer, so we'll quit
sending them.* All of a sudden, the negative thoughts and
feelings are gone. I've had so many people try this one
little practice and say, "I couldn't believe it. I've had these

negative thoughts and feelings all my life. All of a sudden, they stopped." That's one powerful way you can support yourself in changing your downstream thoughts and feelings as your memories heal.

If you find the Memory Engineering Technique and/ or the Autostreaming version is not delivering the results you want, you have two more options: adding an energy medicine booster to either version of the technique (which can up to double its effectiveness), and adding the Healing Codes II process, which addresses the same issues from a different angle while magnifying the effects of both. I'll show you how to do both in the next chapter.

CHAPTER TEN

The Healing Codes II: Energy Tools to Unlock the Door

Although the Memory Engineering Technique is a form of energy medicine itself, it can also be enhanced with additional energy medicine tools.

Some people have an easier time than others accessing their source memories through their image maker. If you find yourself standing at the door of your memories, and it feels like there's a lock on the door, this chapter will show you how to use another set of tools that can help you crack that lock. Once you get inside, you'll be able to access and reengineer your memories a lot more easily.

The Healing Codes II are additional energy tools that can help accelerate the downstream effects of changing the internal memory, so that your thoughts, emotions, feelings, beliefs, behaviors, and physiology can change more quickly.

The Healing Codes are what I am most known for. They were discovered eighteen years ago. You don't have to know what the Healing Codes are to use the tools in this chapter, but in case you're curious, they are a form of energy medicine that uses hand positions to send energy to key centers in the body, primarily to heal the source of health issues.

I am told by experts in the field that the Healing Codes are the number two energy psychology modality in the world. We have clients in fifty states and 172 countries. I am also told our company is the largest practice of its kind in the world, and it's virtually all from word of mouth. I have been interviewed on most network and cable news channels, Oprah.com, PBS, etc.

I have found my clients in Germany, Switzerland, and Austria to strongly value being intellectual, logical, and precise, and the Healing Codes system is still growing in those countries like wildfire—more than anywhere else. Why? It allows you to bypass the conscious mind. If you're intellectually intelligent or lean toward being controlling, adding this kind of energy tool could be the boost that works for you. This was my wife's experience—she is incredibly intelligent, and her mind kept working against her efforts to heal her depression. The Healing Codes were the only thing that worked. But don't worry if you don't think of yourself as intellectual or controlling; they'll be effective in either case.

The Healing Codes II are similar to the first Healing Codes, but they have a completely different purpose. While the Memory Engineering Technique helps *nonphysically* heal your memories using your image maker, the Healing Codes II helps *physically* heal your unconscious, subconscious, and conscious memories—all three at the same time—in a complementary way. According to my testing, the Healing Codes II are about 50 percent more powerful than the original codes, and simpler.

THE HEALING CODES II HAND POSITIONS

The Healing Codes II system focuses on three healing areas:

1. **The brainstem.** The brainstem area is at the center of the base of the skull, right where the skull meets the soft tissue of your neck. This position stimulates your brainstem, or subconscious and unconscious mind.
2. **Prefrontal cortex.** This is your forehead area, about an inch above where the eyebrows would meet if they were to grow together. This position stimulates the prefrontal cortex and everything it's connected to, especially the conscious mind.
3. **The belly button.** This area is directly under the belly button. This position stimulates the gastrointestinal system, where the majority of your immune system is, including the critical microbiome.

To activate these healing areas, simply place your palm over the brainstem, on the forehead (prefrontal cortex), or below the belly button. While holding your hand in this position, I would recommend slow, deep breaths from your stomach, not your chest. (Chest breathing is stress breathing.) Just relax and let your mind and body go, or think of a happy, loving memory. If it feels good to you, focus on the problem and watch it change. Whatever feels right to you is typically the best for this position.

Many people ask how long they should hold the positions, or what results they can expect. Because the Healing Code II works on source issues rather than symptoms, you may not notice any change immediately. People experience a wide range of tangible and intangible results. Some feel euphoria, some feel calmness, and some feel that something has changed but they cannot identify what it is yet. Some feel hope, some experience the diminishing of a negative thought or feeling, and some feel a release of physical pain or tension. A very few (approximately 10 percent of the population) may feel worse before they feel better, which is known as a "healing crisis" or Herxheimer's reaction. Whatever you experience is right for you, but it may be different from anyone else's experience. For that reason, I've given some time suggestions below, but always feel free to hold the positions longer or shorter than recommended.

THE PRIMARY LIFE CODES

On their own, the Healing Codes II is a set of five Primary Life Codes addressing five different aspects of life. When you do them in this order, you can work on any issue you choose and address it from all angles.

1. Primary Life Code 1 addresses negative thoughts, feelings, and beliefs. We want to transform those negative thoughts, feelings, and beliefs from darkness to light, fear to love, falsehood to truth, health issues to health.
2. Primary Life Code 2 addresses illness, disease, and dysfunction—not the symptoms, but the source.

3. Primary Life Code 3 aims to transform fear-based actions and behaviors, pain-based actions and behaviors, addictions, and habits into positive, love-based actions and behaviors.
4. Primary Life Code 4 addresses nonphysical pain (such as mental, emotional, or spiritual pain).
5. Primary Life Code 5 is for any kind of physical pain.

To use the five Primary Life Codes, think of the issue that bothers you most right now—for example, anger at your coworker. Then you can go through all of five Primary Life Codes in order, addressing whatever is related to that issue, known or unknown.

Primary Life Code 1: Negative Thoughts, Feelings, and Beliefs

• Identify the negative thought, feeling, or belief related to your primary issue. For the issue of anger, your negative feeling might be, *I feel like I want to hurt someone.*

• Rate the intensity from 0 to 10.

• Find an earlier memory with the same negative thought and feeling. For example, *At age five, I had a temper tantrum.*

• Rate the intensity of that memory from 0 to 10.

• Pray or ask to become aware of any known or unknown negative memory and physical issue related to this negative thought, feeling, or belief (I want to hurt someone, the temper tantrum, and the anger issue).

- Do the Primary Life Code 1 sequence: *place your left hand on your brainstem, and your right hand on your prefrontal cortex.* While holding your hands in these positions, take slow, deep breaths from your stomach.
- After 15 to 60 seconds, alternate the hands: *left hand prefrontal cortex; right hand brainstem.*
- While doing the code, you can think about whatever you are comfortable with. You can think about the issue itself, the issue of healing, or divine light changing the lie into the truth. You can also simply relax.
- Do the hand positions lightly and gently; there is no need to press hard.
- Timing: You can alternate your hands every 15 to 60 seconds, for however long you want.

Primary Life Code 2: Illness, Disease, and Dysfunction

For the same primary issue (e.g., anger), identify any illness, disease, or dysfunction you feel is related to your issue. For example, *I think this ulcer might be related to this anger issue.*

- Identify the negative thought, feeling, or belief related to this illness, disease, or dysfunction. For example, *this ulcer is physically painful, and it brings with it a sense of hopelessness, as having ulcers is a condition that runs in the family.*
- Find an earlier memory with the same negative thought and feeling. For example, *I also felt hopeless when I got behind in school and felt I couldn't keep up.*
- Pray or ask to become aware of any other known or unknown negative memory and physical issue

related to this illness, disease, or dysfunction (the ulcer, hopelessness, and the anger issue).

• Do the Primary Life Code 2 sequence: *left hand on brainstem (right hand relaxes in your lap).* While holding your hand in this position, take slow, deep breaths from your stomach.

• While doing the code, you can focus on whatever feels comfortable. You can think about the issue itself, focus on the issue healing, or visualize a divine light changing the lie into the truth. You can also simply relax.

• One position only.

• Timing: approximately 1 minute.

Primary Life Code 3: Negative Actions or Behavior

For the same primary issue (e.g., anger), identify a negative action or behavior you feel is related to that issue. For example, *I am drinking too much so I can forget about my anger.*

• Identify the negative thought, feeling, or belief related to this negative action or behavior. For example, *I feel shame or guilt about drinking too much.*

• Find an earlier memory with the same negative thought and feeling. For example, *I felt shame or guilt when I was caught stealing candies from the store.*

• Pray or ask to become aware of any other known or unknown negative memory and physical issue related to this negative action or behavior (drinking too much, shame or guilt, the anger issue).

• Do the Primary Life Code 3 sequence: *right hand on prefrontal cortex (left hand relaxes in your lap).* While holding your hands in this position, take slow, deep breaths from your stomach.

• While doing the code, you can think about whatever you are comfortable with. You can think about the issue itself, the issue of healing, or divine light changing the lie into the truth. You can also simply relax.

• One position only.

• Timing: approximately 1 minute.

Primary Life Code 4: Non-physical Pain (Mental, Emotional, or Spiritual Pain)

For that same primary issue (e.g., anger), identify a non-physical pain related to that issue. For example, *I feel remorse*.

• Identify the negative thought, feeling, or belief related to this nonphysical pain. For example, *I feel I'm not good enough*.

• Find an earlier memory with the same negative thought and feeling. For example, *I felt I wasn't good enough when my boyfriend/girlfriend broke up with me*.

• Pray or ask to become aware of any other known or unknown negative memory and physical issue related to this non-physical pain (remorse, not feeling good enough, and the anger issue).

• Do the Primary Life Code 4 sequence: *Left hand on belly button (right hand relaxes in your lap)*. Note: Placing your hand below your belly button works fine over clothes; it does not have to be on bare skin. While holding your hand in this position, take slow, deep breaths from your stomach.

- While doing the code, you can think about whatever you are comfortable with. You can think about the issue itself, the issue of healing, or divine light changing the lie into the truth. You can also simply relax.
- One position only.
- Timing: approximately 1 minute.

Primary Life Code 5: Physical Pain

For that same primary issue (e.g., anger), identify a physical pain related to that issue. For example, *I have a hangover.*

- Identify the negative thought, feeling, or belief related to this physical pain. For example, *because of the hangover, I feel inadequate to go through the day.*
- Find an earlier memory with the same negative thought and feeling. For example, *I felt inadequate when my mom got sick and I could not help her.*
- Pray or ask to become aware of any other known or unknown negative memory and physical issue related to this physical pain (the hangover, feeling inadequate, and the anger issue).
- Do the Primary Life Code 5 sequence. *Left hand on physical pain area (right hand relaxed in lap).* While holding your hand in this position, take slow, deep breaths from your stomach.
- If you cannot reach the pain area with your left hand, continue position 4: left hand on the belly button, while focusing positive attention on the pain area.

• If you did move your hand to the pain spot, go back to putting your left hand on the belly button, and hold that for a time.

• Alternate your left hand between belly button position and pain area (if you can), ideally until the pain is gone or at least lessened.

• Timing: approximately 1 minute (or longer, if you alternated positions 4 and 5).

USING THE HEALING CODE II WITH THE MEMORY ENGINEERING TECHNIQUE

If you want to give the Memory Engineering Technique a turbo-boost, you can simply add the position of left hand brainstem and right hand prefrontal cortex for thirty seconds, and then left hand prefrontal cortex and right hand brainstem for thirty seconds, alternating as you create each of the six memories. Adding the energy medicine booster turns the Memory Engineering Technique into a mind-body-spirit healing modality: you involve the body with the booster positions, you involve the conscious mind as you create the memories, and you involve your spirit as you address the spiritual issues in your unconscious memories, like forgiveness, love versus fear, rejection, self-worth, and identity. Addressing all three areas gives you the best chance for full healing over the long term.

You can add these booster positions to either the original version or the Autostreaming version. Don't worry about counting seconds; just keep reversing those positions as it feels comfortable throughout the Memory Engineering Technique you learned in the previous chapter.

Here is a step-by-step process you can follow if you're using the original version of the Memory Engineering Technique:

1. Name your issue: What's bothering you?
2. What is the biggest negative feeling you have related to that issue? Rate it from 0 to 10.
3. Understand you can't have a negative feeling without a memory or picture causing it. This process will heal that feeling, and the issue, at the source.
4. What memory or picture comes to mind when you think about this negative emotion? If it's helpful to you, fill out the worksheet to rate and include all parts of the memory, including the thoughts, feelings, beliefs, circumstances, relationships, etc. that are connected to it. If you're one of the few who can't visualize, just say in detail what you feel, and work with the picture that comes from that. No need to use the worksheet.

Here's how to create the six new memories in conjunction with the Healing Code II. You'll be creating four for programming, and two for accuracy. Before each memory, begin by praying to God for a miraculous intervention (if you're comfortable with that) and talking to your heart as a partner in your healing.

5. Programming Memory 1: For the picture or memory you identified, imagine a positive version of the events, where this negative memory never occurred, and instead something happened that made you feel very happy and secure. Imagine it in detail, and live in the memory until you feel the positive feelings and thoughts as if it's happening to you right now.

6. While you continue to look at the new positive picture of the past, pray/ask that the picture become stronger and add the Healing Code II sequence: left hand on brainstem and right hand on prefrontal cortex for about 30 seconds, and then reverse positions as long as it's comfortable, until you really feel the effects of the memory.

7. Programming Memory 2: Create a miraculous version of this same positive past memory, in which you include as much detail as you possibly can.

8. While you continue to look at the new miraculous picture of the past, use the Healing Code II sequence, and pray/ask that the picture become stronger, until you feel the positive effects.

9. Programming Memory 3: Create a new positive memory of the present, based on the new miraculous past memory you created. If that miraculous past memory happened, what would your present look like? Make the

picture detailed enough so that you can feel it right now.

10. While you continue to look at your new miraculous picture of the present, use the Healing Code II sequence, and pray/ask that the picture become stronger, until you feel the positive effects.

11. Programming Memory 4: Create a new memory of the future, based on the new miraculous past memory and present memory you created. If those past and present memories happened, what would your most positive future look like?

12. While you continue to look at your new positive picture of the future, use the Healing Code II sequence, and pray/ask that the picture become stronger, until you feel the positive effects.

13. Default Memory 1: Create a new positive memory of the past in which you don't change what happened, but you change your interpretation of what happened from negative to positive.

14. While you continue to look at your new positive picture of the past, use the Healing Code II sequence, and pray/ask that the picture become stronger, until you feel the positive effects.

15. Default Memory 2: Let go of control, and ask your heart to create the perfect, most

powerful memory for this issue. Ask that it might be the ultimate default memory for this issue whether you ever see it and know what it is or not.

16. If you can see your ultimate default memory, use the Healing Code II sequence, and pray/ask that the picture become stronger, until you feel the positive effects. If not, no problem.

17. When all six memories are complete, rate the overall issue again from 0 to 10. If the issue is still bothering you, you can repeat the process straight away, or repeat it later, until the issue no longer bothers you.

CHAPTER ELEVEN

Memory Engineering in Action

I've seen the Memory Engineering Technique work for almost any issue—health, finances, relationships, anxiety, abuse, addiction—you name it. Here are just a few examples.

CANCER: ERIC'S STORY

One of my clients, Eric, had liver cancer, which many people view as a virtual death sentence. In fact, it was close to my heart because that's what my mother died of in 1988. He got advice from all kinds of people and decided not to go the standard medicine route. He didn't think it would save him anyway, from what he knew. He wanted to feel good for his family during his last year or so.

What happened once he started working with me was extraordinary. He had not been aware of this when we started, but we discovered a memory of anger from when he was a very young child—probably not long after birth. That anger seemed to come from a feeling of rejection, but he didn't have the first clue why. "Of course, I've had a few things happen," he told me, "but nothing that I would even remotely call a trauma." As I learned more about Eric's story, I discovered that he was one of six children. Growing up, he felt like the outcast of the family. He believed that his dad had never really loved him. He never spent as much time with Eric as he did with the other kids, and whatever Eric did was never good enough for his dad.

He eventually remembered more details about his early anger memory: he had been wearing a diaper, he had felt absolutely crushed about himself, and it had something to do with his dad. From that moment on, he patterned his life to do whatever it would take to get his dad's love and respect. When he was about eight years old, he decided the best thing he could possibly do was to become a medical doctor.

Well, he became a medical doctor, and by the time he was in his late twenties, he had built a huge, successful practice in California. He thought, *Now is the time—I can go home, and my dad will finally respect me.*

But when Eric went home to visit his family, there was no change in their relationship. His dad still seemed to act as if he didn't like Eric. All that time he had spent becoming a medical doctor, and it made no difference. He was devastated.

He kept trying, though: Eric accumulated all sorts of accomplishments and awards, bought his parents expensive items they had wanted, was the subject of articles in the paper—but nothing worked. After about ten years, he gave up. He became addicted to drugs, alcohol, and pornography to cope with the pain and became absolutely miserable.

Then, when Eric was in his forties, his dad died. He experienced that as a major trauma, a mixture of intense anger and absolute despair. Now he could never earn his dad's respect. He had failed at his life vow.

About a year after that, he was diagnosed with liver cancer.

When we worked together, we never addressed the cancer. We only addressed his memories: beginning with the most recent, when his dad died, all the way back to when he was in diapers. We worked on every one of those negative memories until they no longer bothered him. We also worked on his interpretation of what the cancer meant to him.

Eric started feeling much better. His fear went away, and he was at peace with dying. Lo and behold, he steadily got better, until about a year and a half later he was declared cancer-free. He'd never had any medical treatment for it, but he had used the extraordinary power of his mind to activate his body's healing abilities.

I believe, and so did he, that it was from the memory engineering. But the real surprise came later, when Eric discovered another source of the anger. It turns out that Eric had a twin. As he was trying to figure out where the memory of anger and rejection came from, he asked his parents a lot of questions. They finally confessed that they weren't expecting two children, and they did not feel that they could financially raise both. He was the one they kept, and they gave up the sibling for adoption.

Well, if you do any research at all, you know that twins are connected like nobody's business. Even if they don't consciously know they are a twin, part of them does. So, in addition to the issues of anger and rejection with his dad, he had the feeling of rejection from being separated from his sibling, which also caused anger. All of this was unconscious, but eventually it leaked up into the conscious.

When he healed both of those issues, his immune system started working much more powerfully because the stress was gone. It healed the liver cancer, which supposedly could not be healed—especially not without treatment, and most probably not even with that, as was the case with my mother.

What started out as liver cancer turned into the most wonderful time of his life. Not only was he healed of the cancer, but he was also able to reconnect with his sibling after all those years.

CAREER: JESSICA'S STORY

Jessica's main issues had to do with success, failure, and finances. She was in her thirties and positive that she was being held down in her career because she was a woman. She went from company to company and job to job. In every one of them, she felt deeply discriminated against, even though she admitted she couldn't point to anything specific.

She said, "I just know I'm being held down because of my sex, because I'm way better than everybody else here!" I started working with her on memory engineering. I don't typically ask clients what they see when I walk them through the process, and in this case, she didn't tell me what she was thinking or feeling. But eventually, she did tell me that she didn't feel she was being held back in her career anymore. The issue no longer bothered her. What she felt now was, "Well, I've gotten some bad breaks, and maybe I am being discriminated against. But even if I am, there's nothing I can do about that, so I'm just going to let that go and work as hard as I can. Whatever happens happens."

Her mind-set had completely shifted. I asked her, "Do you still believe you've been discriminated against?"

"Well, I think so," she answered. "But I'm not angry about it anymore, and I've decided to focus on things that I have control over. I'm not going to ruin my life, my marriage, and my kids, even if it is true."

Jessica went out with this new attitude and immediately got not one raise, but two raises in a four-month period of time, which had never happened in that company before.

Afterward, she talked to her mom about the discrimination issue for the first time. Much to her surprise, her mom told her that during her career, she had outsold everyone at her company for years. She was the top salesperson every single month. But for some reason, only the men got promoted. She had asked about it a couple of times, and they made up some excuse.

"You know what?" her mother told her. "That was when I was pregnant with you."

Her mother had been very upset at the time, thinking,

Okay, I'm bringing a child into the world. I'm going to have a lot more expenses, and I should be able to very comfortably provide—but not if they keep me down at the lowest pay no matter what I do!

"During the time that I was pregnant with you," her mother told her, "I was very angry about being discriminated against financially because I was a woman."

She even apologized, saying, "That obviously somehow impacted you, and I am so sorry for that. Very shortly after that, I quit work altogether because your dad was doing so well, and I wanted to be a stay-at-home mom anyway. It was really never an issue for me ever again."

Although we don't always need to know why we're experiencing an issue in order to heal from it, in Jessica's case it helped her tremendously. Many of us have an inherent need to understand why something is happening to us, or we'll end up making up a reason—which is often wrong and will therefore spike our stress. Now Jessica understood why she felt the way she did and was at peace.

If there are people in your life who were close to your family before you were born, or who may have observed your early childhood, there could be value in reaching out to them to talk. Like Jessica, or many of the other people I've written about in the book, you may find your family history contains answers to questions that you have about your life. Even if you don't have access to direct family information, researching your family's history through census records, immigration ledgers, and other resources may uncover surprising source memories that help you better understand yourself and your path.

Even if you discover something that creates stress short-term, such as the realization that you may not have been wanted as a child, I have found that the truth always sets you free, if you deal with it in love, regardless of others' past or present actions.

RELATIONSHIPS: ELIZABETH'S STORY

I had another client, Elizabeth, who kept getting into relationships with wild men, or men she called "bad boys." She had been divorced twice and was in another relationship with—guess who? A bad boy. She asked me, "Why do I keep repeating this pattern? How come I'm always attracted to these guys who tell me they're going to change for me? I buy it, they don't change, and then it starts all over again!"

What she discovered had to do with the first ten years of her life, when she had been a Mennonite.

She had nothing negative to say about Mennonites, except that she remembered being taught, "You've got to be careful, because people of different faiths just live any way and every way." What came across to her was that people of other faiths were bad people.

Now, here's the kicker. On weekends, they would ride into town in their horse and carriage, dressed in very conservative clothes, and all day she would hear, "You can't do this, you can't do that, and you can't do the other." She would see the other kids in town having so much fun, eating candy and ice cream, and wearing pretty clothes with all kinds of vibrant colors.

When she went into town, those people were nice to her. They didn't seem bad. She started thinking, *I don't see what's so wrong. Maybe what I need is to be bad—at least in the way my family is talking about.*

So she started wanting relationships with what she defined as "bad men." They actually weren't really bad; they just lived differently than the very conservative way she grew up.

When she was ten, her family left that community and started living in the outside world. By then, she was programmed to want relationships with colorful, flamboyant, "bad" men. It ended up backfiring on her, because she absolutely did get into relationships with men who mistreated her.

When we worked through that issue with memory engineering, that desire disappeared. Now she just wanted a nice man who was kind, good, gentle, compassionate, and honest—and that was the next relationship she had.

GRIEF: SUSAN'S STORY

One of my clients, Susan, had trouble emotionally connecting with the people closest to her. Ever since she was a child, she told me, she had always felt disassociated not just from those around her, but even from herself. She had a deep belief that she was alone in life and that everything was up to her, but she couldn't pinpoint where that belief came from. It seemed to be something she was born with.

She had grown up in a two-parent household, where her

father worked outside the home and her mother stayed home with her and her sister. Her mother was extremely engaged and available to her growing up, and she remembered having lots of friends and family members around. She had no memory of abuse or significant loss—at least, nothing more than anyone else she knew. Yet she could not seem to connect to or feel emotionally engaged with her family.

Later that belief of being alone played itself out in her life. She would easily make friends, but her friendships never lasted. She married a man who loved her unconditionally, but she had trouble receiving that love. She chose a job where she worked long hours alone at a computer all day, with little time or energy left over for her husband, children, home, relationships, or anything. She created a life where she was indeed alone.

She didn't want to live this way. She felt terribly guilty about neglecting everything she valued most, but she didn't know how to change it.

We worked on the issue of feeling alone with the Memory Engineering Technique. When we got to the sixth step, where we allowed the heart to create a new default memory, she told me that she saw an image of herself trapped in a dark basement full of skeletons.

We began again with the Memory Engineering Technique, using that image as the presenting issue. When I asked her what she saw when she imagined that basement full of skeletons as a positive image, she said that she saw the skeletons, one by one, transform into family members who had died, who recognized her and greeted her.

I had already known from her family history that a

number of people had died young and tragically. On her father's side, both her great-grandfathers and her grandfather had died in their twenties, and on her mother's side, the last three generations had each lost a young child. But she never thought much about it, because she hadn't personally known any of these family members.

She hadn't realized that her feeling of disassociation and her belief that she was alone came from multiple generations of unexpressed grief, until her heart showed her that image. When it did, she knew instantly that it was indeed the source of her issue.

When she created the miraculous memory, she saw herself at a big, lively dinner table, surrounded by all the family members who had died young, now grown to adulthood, healthy, laughing, and with spouses and children of their own. She said she had never felt so happy and connected.

The wonderful thing about this miraculous memory was that she believed it was also partially true. She believed all her family members were still spiritually alive in some way, and she could connect with them in her mind at any time. She believed she would see them again when she passed away as well.

The result is that she no longer feels alone. Rather than being sources of fear and abandonment, memories of her deceased family members are now consciously and unconsciously a source of love and support. She has lessened her work responsibilities so she can be more available to her family, and she feels much more connected to her life and her community.

ANXIETY: JOHN'S STORY

John was the stereotypical "guy's guy": big, strong, jovial, friendly, someone easy to hang out with.

John was also a worrier. He had a great job, but all of a sudden he started having pain in his arms, forearms, and hands, to the point that it affected his work. He was diagnosed with carpal tunnel syndrome. It kept getting worse and worse, until finally one day he came in to see me with both arms in casts. Doctors were trying to immobilize his arms to let them heal. We started addressing the issue through memory engineering, focusing on the issue of worrying instead of his medical symptoms.

He had a very specialized job, and if he lost that job, he felt he couldn't just go out and get another one. Fortunately, his job was specialized around the one thing he was really good at, at the only company around that did it. That made his fears even worse. He said, "My kids are in school here. They're happy. My wife grew up here; she does not want to move. Our whole life is here. If I lose this job—first of all, I won't be able to get any other job like this if the carpal tunnel doesn't get better—and even if it does get better, I can't come close to matching my current salary without us moving somewhere far away."

That really magnified the worry and the resistance and made it even harder to break through.

One day, it all clicked for him. He was sitting with his eyes closed while I was leading him through a meditation. He opened his eyes, almost in a startled way, and said, "It just changed." I said, "What?" He said, "It just changed." He kept saying that: "It just changed. I can't believe it changed." I said, "What changed, John?" Finally, he said, "The worry is gone."

We had focused on changing and editing memories for weeks, and he had been doing it at home on his own in between meetings. For whatever reason, after who knows how many hours of creating and editing memories, he had gotten to the source and changed it, because his worrying was gone. In a very short period of time, his carpal tunnel went away completely. As far as I know, he lived happily ever after.

The issue was never the carpal tunnel, although of course that's what he thought. The issue was the memories inside of him—and we never found out what memories were at the source, or at least I didn't. We were able to fix them by essentially taking out one software package and putting in another without knowing exactly what memories were the problem. Now, it took some time and effort. I guarantee you, there was a period of several weeks when he thought we were making no progress at all. Then all of a sudden, the issue was gone.

Note: These are very specific examples of actual clients for whom we knew or found out the history related to the problem and its underlying memories. I have had just as many clients who did not know their own history or where the problem came from. And sometimes no amount of searching turns up any relevant answers. No problem! Just begin the Memory Engineering Technique with the "free floating" or "circumstantial" negative feelings and thoughts until (1) the underlying feelings and thoughts change, and (2) the physical symptoms change and/or go away.

I want to say one more thing about John's issue. Many people think they're living a life of meaning and purpose by just slogging through life, because they're doing it for the people they love—not realizing that the quality of their experience is actually part of a meaningful and purposeful life.

Not only that, they're also teaching the people they love that life is not really about experiencing meaning and purpose. It's about just doing your duty and getting through it for the people you care about. I would agree that's better than becoming a serial killer. But still, at the end of your life, you're going to look back and say, "Well, it could have been worse, but you know, I sure felt like something was missing."

That's how John felt. He had a good job. He was a nice guy. His life wasn't horrible. He truly believed he was doing the best he could to be responsible and that he was living a life of meaning and purpose because he was doing his best for his family.

Then that injury came up. What if he had decided to just hunker down and deal with it, maybe with surgery, instead of dealing with the source? He would never have freed himself from the worry that had been weighing him down.

After our work together, John didn't radically overhaul his life. He didn't quit his job, leave his family, and go open a surf shop in some tropical paradise. But he did change his perspective on his work and his role. He was able to let go of the fear that he was only good at one thing and that his entire life would be defined by work that didn't even mean very much him. He changed his perspective in a way that allowed him to work as well as he had been, but without putting as much pressure on himself. He only changed the way he viewed his internal memories and therefore his current circumstances.

Remember what Dr. Jimmy Netterville wrote on his napkin: there is so much we don't know, and we have a track record of condemning new things that years later become mainstream and accepted. If it obviously works for most people, and does no harm, try it! That's all I am asking of you.

EPILOGUE

Programmed for Miracles

In counseling, I often ask people, "Have you ever felt you were special, that you were supposed to live an extraordinary life?" About eight out of ten people say yes. "Yeah. When I was a kid, yeah..." I think that's part of why we pretend to be superheroes when we're little.

Why don't we pretend to be superheroes when we're forty-five (well, most of us, anyway)? Sure, one reason is simply maturity. But I believe a bigger reason is that most of us have lost hope. We've so gotten used to the path of fear that hopelessness and survival mode have become our new normal. I also believe that feeling of being special and belief in an extraordinary life is still there! That's why the recent Marvel and DC movies have been so big—they activate that "anything is possible" belief that has been in us since childhood.

When people have a turnaround in their life, those around them will very often say, "What's happened to you? You seem almost like a little kid again." Why do they say "little kid"? Because they've gotten some of that special feeling back. They're trying, even at forty-five, to go back and take action on that call to be extraordinary they've been denying for twenty-five years.

When we come into this world, our minds, bodies, and souls are programmed to survive. But I believe we also have a hidden encrypted file within us that can allow us to be extraordinary. When we get to the age at which we know the moral difference between right and wrong, if we're not in a constantly life-threatening situation, that encrypted file opens.

Now we are still made to survive, but we also have a calling to be extraordinary. To become extraordinary, to allow that encrypted file to run your programming, takes something that most people would say is abnormal. Others would call it miraculous. It is this: *you have to let go of the compulsion to survive.* You must choose a life of love rather than a life of survival.

Survival is rooted in fear. When we're born, our brain is in a delta-theta brainwave state for the only time in our life. It's much more geared toward fear and stays there until that encrypted file opens. Until then, that's just the way it is—there's nothing we can do about it except survive, learn, and grow.

But once that second file opens and we shift out of delta-theta, and then we have a choice every day for the rest of our lives. We don't have to accept the call to be extraordinary. We're free to reject it. Although if we do, we'll probably still sense that call from time to time for the rest of our life. If we continue to reject it, later in life we'll feel like we've missed something.

When we choose love with all of our heart and let go of seeking pleasure and avoiding pain with all of our heart (and our heart knows whether we've really done that or not), that file becomes our new software, and we experience what was never possible before. In a way, we start living like a superhero.

Love opens the door to the miraculous. It leads to a life of grace.

What do I mean by a life of grace? Grace is more than just internal love for yourself. Grace is internal *and* external love. It means being in right relationship not just with yourself, but with everyone else around you, including the Source of the universe, or God.

In fact, to fully experience the possibilities of grace, I believe you have to be in right relationship with God or your Higher Power. It is not the purpose of this book to tell you my beliefs about this, but I do believe that right relationship is what taps you into the full power of the supernatural.

The system of grace is the exact opposite of the system of law. The system of law goes by many different names: the law of cause and effect, Newton's Third Law of Motion (every action has an equal and opposite reaction), the Law of Attraction, karma, "you reap what you sow." But they're all really the same law: what you get depends on what you do.

Those laws are absolutely real, and they produce real results. But their results are limited. There is an even higher system that is completely different from any of

262 ▸ *The Memory Code*

those laws and any other law I've heard of. It's called grace. It results in experiencing your highest potential, because grace connects you to the supernatural. It does not follow the rules of classical physics or any known laws that govern the universe. It miraculously changes your have-tos into want-tos and produces the best results for you *and* everyone else long term.

In my experience, most people don't really understand grace. They think it's synonymous with forgiveness, or getting something for free. It's neither. It's never having something to forgive in the first place. And it's not free—it's paid for by the offended party, not the offending party.

To illustrate, I'd like to share a few stories.

A STORY OF GRACE

It was Paul's sixteenth birthday, and he woke up more excited than on any Christmas that he could remember. His mom and dad had consented to let him miss the first couple hours of school so that he could go take his driver's test that morning, as soon as the DMV opened.

Sure enough, he arrived before they even unlocked the doors, and when they did, Paul went bounding into the driver testing center. The workers got a kick out of how excited he was, although they'd seen it many times before.

Paul had all the necessary paperwork already filled out. He signed his name, and then his dad signed, attesting that Paul was really who his birth certificate said he was. Then Paul was ushered over to a machine to take the written test.

After about thirty minutes, Paul was done and was told that he had passed, only missing one question, which did not surprise his father since Paul had been studying for about six weeks. He got a big kick out of the fact that Paul was reacting to getting his license almost exactly the way he had when he was a kid.

Next was the road test. He could see some perspiration on Paul's forehead as they went out to his dad's six-year-old Oldsmobile Cutlass Supreme, which Paul had also been practicing in, not for six weeks, but probably for six months.

Paul did everything right. When they got back, the highway patrol lady said he did an excellent job. Paul grinned from ear to ear. They went back inside, and after about fifteen minutes, Paul was given his first driver's license. His parents had gotten him a ten-year-old used Chevrolet to drive. Paul was absolutely tickled and felt freedom like he had never felt in his life.

About three months later, Paul's dad brought a huge surprise home: a brand-new, shiny red Corvette.

Paul could not believe it. He knew immediately that it wasn't for him, but he still couldn't believe it. They'd never had a car like this. They usually bought their cars secondhand to save some money.

When his dad got out of the car, Paul went running up to him, and his mom came out of the house to give his dad a hug. They explained the situation. It had always been his dad's dream to have a red Corvette, for as long as he could remember. He'd never been able to afford one, and really couldn't now, but he'd been saving money for about ten years in order to get this car and fulfill his lifelong dream.

Paul got in and saw what it felt like to sit in the driver's seat. It was the coolest thing he'd ever seen. It was one of those moments for the family that would be forever frozen in time.

About three months after that, Paul had gotten up his courage to ask out the girl he'd had a crush on for the last five years. To his delight and amazement, she said yes. Overjoyed, Paul went to his dad and asked to borrow the Corvette. He didn't really think the answer would be yes, but thought he'd take a shot. He was convinced this girl was the one for him, so he thought it was worth it, for first impression's sake.

He could imagine how the night would go if he somehow got a yes, so he went to his dad and blurted it out. "Dad, I finally got a date with April." His dad hugged him. His mom heard, and she came in and hugged him, too. They clapped and whooped and made a big deal. Paul thought, *If I'm ever going to do it, this is the time.*

"Dad, is there any way you would let me borrow your Corvette for my first date with April?"

Dad looked at Mom; Mom looked at Dad. They consulted each other without speaking. There were a couple of nods, and his dad said, "Okay, son." Paul absolutely could not believe it. He knew this was going to be the best night of his life and was more excited than he could ever remember being.

The night came, and his dad just said, "Be careful." His son was an excellent driver, so he didn't really give him the third degree. He just said, "Be careful. Have a great time." His mom said, "Now, you drive slow. You know that thing goes way faster than your old car." He said, "I know, Mom. I'll be careful," and off he went.

The night was fabulous, wonderful, and every other

adjective that Paul could've imagined. They went to dinner and a movie, where he got his nerve up to hold her hand. His hand had started sweating profusely, but he didn't care, and she didn't seem to care, either. He took her home and even got a kiss on the cheek at the end of the night. She said she would like to do it again. How could it have gone any better?

On the way home, Paul was listening to music and singing at the top of his lungs, even though that wasn't one of his greater gifts. Not a care in the world. He came to a curve and—even decades later he had no idea how it happened—he hit the gas instead of the brake. The car was going so fast, and he had no control. Before he even knew it, the curve was gone, and the car was wrapped around a telephone pole.

The first thing he discovered was that he was almost completely unharmed. His left arm was bleeding a little bit, but other than that, he seemed to be untouched by the accident. The door wouldn't open, so he had to crawl out the window. Looking at the car, he just broke down crying. It was totaled.

The police came. They were really kind to him. They could tell he hadn't been drinking, he wasn't on drugs. It was an innocent accident. They called a wrecker service to come and get the car, probably taking it to a dump somewhere. Then they got Paul in the police car to take him home. When they got to the house, the policeman said to him, "Paul, I'm sorry, but this part you've got to do by yourself. Keep your head up, son."

Paul was still fighting tears. He kept thinking of the look on his dad's face when he drove the Corvette home, then hearing over and over in his head that he had been saving for it for ten years.

Paul got out of the car, walked up to the front door, and walked in. Mom and Dad said, "How'd it go?" They'd been waiting all night, talking to each other, giggling, laughing about how excited their son was. His dad was actually really tickled that Paul had his first date in his car. But as soon as they looked at his face, they knew that something had gone wrong.

Mom first said, "Honey, what's wrong?" and rushed up to him, and then Dad, too, asked, "Son, are you okay? What's going on?"

Then Paul dropped the news. "I wrecked the Corvette, and it's totaled."

His dad asked, "Was April okay?"

And Paul said, "Yeah, I had dropped her off before it happened."

"Well, are you okay?"

"Yeah, I've got this little cut here, but it doesn't even need stitches. It's not bad. I'm fine. I'm just..." And then he started into the speech he'd been practicing in the back of the policeman's car. "Dad, I'm just so sorry about your car. I know you saved for ten years. I know you dreamed about that all your life. I'm just so sorry. Can you ever forgive me? I'm hoping and praying that you had it insured."

His dad looked at him with tears in his eyes and said, "Son, it was not insured. I had it insured, but then your mom and I decided to change insurance companies. We just yesterday told the old insurance company, 'Let's go ahead and cancel.' I hadn't gotten around to getting the new insurance yet."

But the tears in his dad's eyes didn't seem to be for the car. He grabbed Paul in a bear hug, picked him up, and said, "Paul, don't you worry about that car. That's just a machine. Don't you worry about that for a second. You're the thing that's important. I love you so much, and I'm just so glad you're okay. Don't you give that car a second thought."

His mom didn't say much of anything. She had gone to get some supplies to patch up his cut. After the family talked a little more, Paul went to his room, still wracked with grief. The car was not insured. His dad saved for that for ten years. There's no way he'd be able to get another one, and it was all his fault.

The next day, Paul was in the yard when his dad drove home, not in a new Corvette, not in a six-year-old Cutlass Supreme, but in a Yugo. At that time, people made jokes about Yugos. They were very small, not very reliable—a huge step down even from the old Cutlass.

But Dad seemed as cheerful as he ever was. "Hey, Paul. How's it going, man? Great to see you. How was your day? How was school?"

Paul said again, "Dad, I'm just so sorry about your car."

"What did I tell you? You don't ever need to say anything again. I don't care about that car. I care about you." Paul hugged him, and Dad hugged him back. Paul went back to shooting baskets in the backyard, and his dad went in the house.

Paul's feelings improved over the next few weeks. He could tell his dad was not putting on an act. He really seemed to be okay with what had happened and didn't blame Paul at all—even though Paul didn't know how that was possible. He tried to put himself in that situation and felt sure he would've blamed his son and probably give him a good scolding and some kind of punishment. He couldn't believe what an incredible dad he had.

Then a few days later, an interesting thing happened. Paul was in the yard as his dad came home, but instead of going into the house to kiss his mother right off, he came to see Paul and said, "Hey, Paul, I got a favor to ask you." So Paul said, "What?" His dad said, "Well, I've got a big business associate coming into town to meet with me tomorrow. I'm supposed to pick him up at the airport, but my car is absolutely filthy. I've still got a whole bunch of studying and work tonight to get ready for this event that my company's been planning for several months. Could you wash my car real quick for me?"

Paul was overjoyed. He had wanted to do something to give back to his dad, to show his dad that he was sorry, to somehow make amends in some small way. Paul leaped at that. "Absolutely. No problem at all. In fact, anytime you want it washed, just let me know and I'll be happy to wash it. No problem, Dad. Happy to do it."

Dad winked at him, smiled, said, "Thanks, son," and went into the house. Paul went into the garage to get the bucket with the cleaning supplies and pull the hose around. Paul washed that car, and he noticed that he was singing again for the first time since the night of his date, and wasn't sure why, because he had never gotten any joy out of washing cars before.

GRACE CHANGES HAVE-TOS INTO WANT-TOS

This is a true story. To me, it is a good illustration of a life of grace. Paul was expecting law. Paul was expecting punishment. Paul was expecting, "You know you're supposed to do this, and not that. You know that you were not supposed to wreck the car. Since you wrecked the car, you're grounded for the next month, or you need to do extra chores, or you need to get a part-time job to help pay for a new car."

What difference do you think it made to Paul that his dad reacted the way he did—without any judgment or consequence at all, even though he "deserved" it?

Paul would tell me, years later, that this was the turning point of his life. Not that his life had been bad before, but this was when he really felt totally, completely loved, valued, and secure as a person of worth, no matter what he did. None of that was dependent on what he did. It was just dependent on Paul being Paul, even with all his mistakes. Whether we realize it or not, that's what all of us really want.

I think most parents would have first made sure that he and April were okay. But after that, even if the father didn't lash out, he probably would have been devastated with his own loss. He had saved for ten years. It had been his lifelong dream. It was probably the only time in his life he would ever be able to afford it, and there was no evidence that I know of that he started saving again. After the Corvette was totaled, I think he gave all that up.

The difference between the normal response and the actual response was a turning point in Paul's life for the good. The accident could have been a major trauma. He

270 The Memory Code

could have been blamed; his father could have been furious, or his mom could have said, "Do you know how long your dad saved for this car? Do you know this has been his dream his entire life? Do you know that it wasn't insured, that we were trusting that you would drive safely, and realize how careful you needed to be?"

But instead, both parents were totally focused on Paul, and that he was not only okay physically, but also emotionally and spiritually. They reacted in a way that preserved their relationship first and foremost.

Now most people wouldn't do that without an enormous amount of effort. They would be so devastated that they would immediately be plunged into stress themselves and therefore think about themselves and their loss. It's certainly understandable, isn't it? When we live under the law system, we can't help but think about how everything is going to affect us, because our survival is the most important thing. But when we are living under the grace system, we are able to experience personal disappointment that isn't all consuming. Whatever our feelings may be, we can feel them while also taking stock of how others are doing. We are able to prioritize what's most crucial and have a reaction that we are proud of that serves the greatest good.

The bottom line is that Paul's dad was never mad; he took in the news of what had happened, and he prioritized what was most crucial—in this case, that Paul and April were safe, and that Paul not come away from the experience with a new emotional scar. As a result of seeing grace given to him, it created a powerful memory for Paul of choosing grace himself. Before, Paul told me he would have grumbled and complained if he had ever been asked to wash someone's car. Afterward, he was actually excited to wash his dad's car! His have-to had changed to a want-to; it just happened, instantly and miraculously.

The event became a powerful memory that Paul would be able to draw on again and again in life, creating a model for him to base his own behavior on in all kinds of situations where a response from the grace system would benefit everyone involved. Paul would say it changed him forever. In other words, the grace-based Paul was a perceptibly different person than the fear/pleasure/pain Paul, not just to others, but, most important, to himself. He continued to apply his father's grace to himself and others for the rest of his life. Many people credited Paul's grace with positive changes in their own lives. This story was told at Paul's funeral, and it illuminated Paul's secret to all the people who suspected he had one.

I believe that Paul's dad understood and lived a life of grace, even if he wouldn't have called it that, and many other people have as well. People all throughout history have figured this out, even if they couldn't explain it in words.

For example, I remember reading my grandmother's diary from the early part of the twentieth century, and I believe she had discovered this way of life as well.

She and my grandfather were living in America as a German family during the Second World War. She went through two traumatic events: first, being mocked and ridiculed by her friends and neighbors because of her German ancestry—even though my grandfather fought for America and won a medal in the war.

Second, they owned and operated a Southern planta-
tion that my grandfather had built. During the Depression, the bank called their loan of $500. They didn't have
that much, so they lost what they had built over many
years of sweat and toil. They had to move to a smaller
house in a different town.

From what I've been told by people who knew her
personally, everyone said the exact same thing: if anyone was an actual living angel from heaven, it was that
woman. Not only did she not return anger for anger, but
she also showed nothing but love. She would bake pies
and visit people who were sick regularly, even people
who didn't like her.

She worked all day every day; if help was needed, she
would be the first one there. Despite cruelty, mocking, and
devastating life circumstances, she appeared to be totally
unaffected. Her diary talked about the joy she had helping
others, and how she loved America and the American people.

My own two brothers have told me that they've never
known anyone else like her. She was unbelievably kind and
loving, and laughed all the time. Whenever anyone else was
around, she was totally focused on and invested in them,
with no thought for herself. I was the baby in the family
and don't remember her at all, and I feel a little jealous of
my brothers when they talk about her.

I'm sure some of you reading this may be living a life
of grace, too; I've had a few of those people in my counseling office. It's just that in my experience, the percentage of
those who figure it out on their own is minuscule, when
all of us have the potential to be experiencing life like that,

and having that kind of effect on our children, our spouses, and ultimately, the world.

I had a similar experience to Paul's, although it happened differently. For example, when I was living under the Law of Externals, there was nothing I hated more than cleaning toilets. It was disgusting; I despised it; I would do anything to get out of it, including lie.

At the same time, we were broke. One way that we made ends meet was that my wife and I were cleaning houses together. Once again, I was cleaning toilets. Sometimes they were absolutely disgusting—but now I was singing and humming and smiling and laughing while I cleaned toilets. I literally felt as if there were nowhere on earth I would rather be than where I was right now. Why? Because my wife was right in the next room. The next time she saw me, she was going to smile at me with that smile that said, "I love you with every fiber of my being"—when six months earlier, she didn't want to be anywhere near me.

It's not that I loved cleaning toilets. It's that I was cleaning toilets in love. It gave me a chance to be with my wife, whom I loved more than anything, and that's what was most important.

Cleaning toilets didn't matter anymore because of the love. That's what grace does. It makes poverty meaningless. It overrides physical pain. It overrides cleaning a nasty, horrible toilet. It overcomes just about anything in your life that you can name.

For Hope, it was football. Whenever she'd walk into the room and a football game was on, she'd screw up her face and say, "I *hate* that. Can you please turn that off?"

After my turnaround (which also had a big effect on her), she'd say, "When's the next football game? I'd really like to go." Why? It wasn't that all of a sudden she loved watching football. She was watching football in love—because she knew I loved it, and she wanted to be with me. It was about the relationship.

You now have a choice to make. Do you want to be extraordinary in your own way? Do you want to change your have-tos to want-tos? Do you want the best part of you to become your default programming, or do you want to continue living in survival mode?

You must decide whether you want to prioritize living by the spiritual or by the natural. Fear, or a life of law, comes from the natural world, from our physical brain and its fight-or-flight mechanisms. Love, or a life of grace, comes from the spiritual world, and therefore has the supernatural power to produce miraculous results you could never achieve through natural willpower.

Love itself doesn't even really make sense from a strictly natural, survival-of-the-fittest perspective. What makes sense in the natural world is seeking pleasure and avoiding pain, not making yourself more vulnerable to pain (which is what real love often requires). What makes sense in the natural world is defining success as getting the end result you want when you want it. Choosing love even when it causes you pain, and choosing to give up what you really want and what you think will make you happy, seems suspicious in the natural world—but not in the supernatural. The practical difference between living according to the natural and the spiritual is like the difference between riding a horse and driving a car, or solving math problems with paper and pencil versus using a calculator.

Both are programmed within you. But choosing love is the only way to put that extraordinary file in the driver's seat.

The bottom line is that the results we all want in our life—love, joy, peace, health, happiness, and success even beyond our own desires—are beyond our physical and mental power to produce. There's only one way to tap into supernatural power to achieve those kinds of results, and that's the choice you have before you right now. Choose the Law of Internals. Choose love. Choose the spiritual. Choose a life of grace. Heal the fear-based memories that are at the true source of your issues. Would you rather spend your energy treating symptoms for the rest of your life or bringing miraculous positive change to yourself, your loved ones, and the world?

I believe you now have the understanding and the tools to start down that path. You have the opportunity to be programmed for miracles. The choice is yours.

ACKNOWLEDGMENTS

To Amanda, Harry, Michael, Steve, Leah, Emily, Jeff, Alana, Alli, and Bernd: I could never have done this without you, and you even made it easy for me. I love you and thank you from the bottom of my heart!

NOTES

Chapter 1: How Humans Were Designed to Function (But Don't Anymore)

1 Caroline Leaf, *Who Switched Off My Brain?* New Edition (Thomas Nelson, 2009).

2 Caroline Leaf, *The Perfect You* (Baker Books, 2017), 52.

3 Rebecca Turner and Margaret Altemus, "Preliminary Research on Plasma Oxytocin in Normal Cycling Women: Investigating Emotion and Interpersonal Distress," *Psychiatry: Interpersonal and Biological Processes*, 62, 2 (July 1999): 97–113.

4 Bruce Lipton, "Are You Programmed at Birth?," www.healyourlife.com/are-you-programmed-at-birth.

5 Ned Herrmann, "What Is the Function of the Various Brainwaves?" *Scientific American*, www.scientificamerican.com/article/what-is-the-function-of-t-1997-12-22/, accessed March 4, 2019.

6 Herrmann, "What Is the Function of the Various Brainwaves?"

7 Lipton, "Are You Programmed at Birth?" www.healyourlife.com/are-you-programmed-at-birth.

8 Herrmann, "What Is the Function of the Various Brainwaves?"

9 Lipton, "Are You Programmed at Birth?" www.healyourlife.com/are-you-programmed-at-birth.

10 Sue Goetinck Ambrose, "A Cell Forgets," *The Dallas Morning News*, October 20, 2004, legacy.sandiegouniontribune.com/uniontrib/20041020/news_z1c20cell.html.

11 Bruce Lipton, *The Biology of Belief* (Hay House, 2008), 89.

12 Sources: Cort A. Pedersen, University of North Carolina, Chapel Hill; Kerstin Uvnäs Moberg, *The Oxytocin Factor: Tapping the Hormone of Calm, Love, and Healing* (Pinter & Martin, 2011).

13 "Curse of the Lottery," *THS Investigates*, E! Entertainment Television, documentary, 120 min., originally aired September 24, 2006.

14 Brent Lambert, "75 Years in the Making: Harvard Just Released Its Epic Study on What Men Need to Live a Happy Life," FEELguide, April 29, 2013, www.feelguide.com/2013/04/29/75-years-in-the-making-harvard-just-released-its-epic-study-on-what-men-require-to-live-a-happy-life/. This article includes a synopsis of the study, but the full findings can be found in George Vaillant, *Triumphs of Experience: The Men of the Harvard Grant Study* (Belknap Press, 2015).

15 Kim Painter, "To Live Longer, Fight Less, Study Shows," *USA Today*, May 12, 2014.

16 See UMass Boston, "Still Face Experiment: Dr. Edward Tronick," YouTube, November 30, 2009, www.youtube.com/watch?v=apzXGEbZht0.

17 Matthew Jones, "11 Billion Reasons The Self Help Industry Doesn't Want You To Know The Truth About Happiness," Inc.com, www.inc.com/matthew -jones/11-billion-reasons-self-help-industry-doesnt-want-you-to-know -truth-about-happiness.html

18 Harvard Health Publishing, "Understanding the Stress Response," www .health.harvard.edu/staying-healthy/understanding-the-stress-response.

Chapter 2: Making Memories

1 Julia Shaw, *The Memory Illusion* (Random House UK, 2016), 67.

2 Jeneen Interlandi, "New Estimate Boosts the Human Brain's Memory Capacity 10-Fold," *Scientific American*, February 5, 2016, www.scientificameri can.com/article/new-estimate-boosts-the-human-brain-s-memory -capacity-10-fold/; Tia Ghose, "The Human Brain's Memory Could Store the Entire Internet," *LiveScience*, February 18, 2016, www.livescience.com/53751 -brain-could-store-internet.html.

3 Steven Pinker, *Enlightenment Now: The Case for Reason, Science, Humanism, and Progress* (Viking, 2018), 48.

4 Lesley Evans Ogden, "How Extreme Fear Shapes What We Remember," BBC Future, February 6, 2015, www.bbc.com/future/story/20150205-how -extreme-fear-shapes-the-mind.

5 Jeff Stibel, "Pessimists: The World Is Better Than You Think. Your Brain Makes You Think Otherwise," *USA Today*, October 23, 2018, www.usatoday .com/story/money/usaandmain/2018/10/23/pessimists-your-brain -tricking-you-into-believing-things-bad/1732155002/.

6 Shaw, *The Memory Illusion*, 38–40.

7 Nathan H. Lents and Deryn Strange, "Trauma, PTSD, and Memory Dis-tortion: Evolution May Be Partly to Blame," *Psychology Today*, May 23, 2016, www.psychologytoday.com/us/blog/beastly-behavior/201605/trauma -ptsd-and-memory-distortion.

8 Julia Shaw, "What Experts Wish You Knew about False Memories," MIND Guest Blog, *Scientific American*, August 8, 2016, blogs.scientificamerican.com/ mind-guest-blog/what-experts-wish-you-knew-about-false-memories/?WT .mc_id=SA_MB_20160810. Also see Leonard Mlodinow, *Subliminal: How Your Unconscious Mind Rules Your Behavior* (Vintage/Random House, 2013), 45.

9 Julia Shaw, "What Experts Wish You Knew about False Memories," MIND Guest Blog, *Scientific American*, August 8, 2016, blogs.scientificamerican .com/mind-guest-blog/what-experts-wish-you-knew-about-false -memories/?WT.mc_id=SA_MB_20160810; Anne Trafton, "Neuroscien-tists Plant False Memories in the Brain," MIT News, July 25, 2013, news.mit .edu/2013/neuroscientists-plant-false-memories-in-the-brain-0725.

10 Julia Shaw, *The Memory Illusion*, Kindle edition, location 204.

11 Judith Shulevitz, "The Science of Suffering: Kids Are Inheriting Their Parents' Trauma; Can Science Stop It?" *New Republic*, November 16, 2014, www.newrepublic.com/article/120144/trauma-genetic-scientists-say -parents-are-passing-ptsd-kids.

12 Rebecca Smith, "Children of Holocaust Survivors 'Learn' Fear from Mothers: Researcher," *The Telegraph*, July 29, 2014, www.telegraph.co.uk/news/health/ news/10995894/Children-of-Holocaust-survivors-learn-fear-from -mothers-researcher.html.

13 Richard Gray, "Phobias May Be Memories Passed Down in Genes from Ancestors," *The Telegraph*, December 1, 2013, www.telegraph.co.uk/news/ science/science-news/10486479/Phobias-may-be-memories-passed -down-in-genes-from-ancestors.html.

14 Esther Landhuis, "How Dad's Stresses Get Passed Along to Offspring," *Scientific American*, November 8, 2018, www.scientificamerican.com/article/how-dads -stresses-get-passed-along-to-offspring/.

15 Eytan Halon, "Israeli Study: Nervous System Can Transmit Messages to Future Generations," *Jerusalem Post*, June 7, 2019, https://www.jpost.com/ Israel-News/Israeli-study-Nervous-system-can-transmit-messages-to-future -generations-591795.

16 Dan M. Kahan, Ellen Peters, Maggie Wittlin, Paul Slovic, Lisa Larrimore Ouellette, Donald Braman, and Gregory Mandel, "The Polarizing Impact of Science Literacy and Numeracy on Perceived Climate Change Risks," *Nature Climate Change* vol. 2 (2012), pp. 732–735, www.nature.com/articles/ nclimate1547.

17 Brendan Nyhan and Jason Reifler, "When Corrections Fail: The Persistence of Political Misperceptions," *Political Behavior*, vol. 32, no. 2 (June 2010), pp. 303–330, full text available at www.dartmouth.edu/~nyhan/nyhan -reifler.pdf. Also see Gordon Pennycook and David Rand, "Why Do People Fall for Fake News?" *New York Times*, January 19, 2019, www.nytimes .com/2019/01/19/opinion/sunday/fake-news.html. The authors, who are psychologists, cite the Kahan and Nyhan-Reifler studies as part of a body of evidence supporting the idea that "our ability to reason is hijacked by our partisan convictions," although based on their own study, they personally believe we're simply intellectually lazy. Either way, I'd still say the underly- ing reason has to do with our memories: if we don't have a fear-based mem- ory related to the issue, we have more access to our reasoning abilities. One very important aspect most studies don't control for is the stress level of their participants, which to me determines everything about how they respond in any situation. If they're not stressed, they have more access to their reason- ing abilities, and vice versa.

Chapter 3: The Devolution of Memory

1 Andrew Weil, *Health and Healing: The Philosophy of Integrative Medicine and Optimum Health* (Houghton Mifflin, 1983), 57.

Chapter 4: The Two Laws

1 Clint Gresham, "Super Bowl Champ: I've Won AND Lost the Big Game—Here's the Incredible Thing I Learned," FoxNews.com, February 2, 2019, www.foxnews.com/opinion/super-bowl-champ-ive-won-and-lost-the-big-game-heres-the-incredible-thing-i-learned.

2 Daniel Gilbert, *Stumbling on Happiness*, Vintage, 2007.

Chapter 5: Why You Can't Do What's Best for You

1 Helen E. Fisher, *Why We Love: The Nature and Chemistry of Romantic Love* (Henry Holt and Co., 2005), 52–53; Mark B. Kastleman, *The Drug of the New Millennium: The Brain Science behind Internet Pornography Use* (Power Think Publishing, 2007). For more on the tidal wave of brain chemicals, see Michael D. Lemonick, "The Chemistry of Desire," *Time*, January 19, 2004, and R. A. Wise, "Dopamine, Learning, and Motivation," *Nature Reviews Neuroscience* 5 (2004), 483–494.

2 Stephen Cave, "There's No Such Thing as Free Will," *The Atlantic*, June 2016, www.theatlantic.com/magazine/archive/2016/06/theres-no-such-thing-as-free-will/480750/.

3 National Geographic, *Your Brain: A User's Guide (100 Things You Never Knew)*. Single issue magazine, 2012.

4 Gaia Vince, "Hacking the Nervous System," Mosaic, May 26, 2015, http://mosaicscience.com/story/hacking-nervous-system; Christopher Bergland, "How Does the Vagus Nerve Convey Gut Instincts to the Brain?" *Psychology Today* online, May 23, 2014, hwww.psychologytoday.com/blog/the-athletes-way/201405/how-does-the-vagus-nerve-convey-gut-instincts-the-brain.

5 Romans 7:19, ESV.

6 Cave, "There's No Such Thing as Free Will."

7 For example, see Kelly McGonigal's *The Upside of Stress* (Avery, 2015).

8 Jenny L. Cook, "How Stress Hits Women's Brains Harder—and Why Men Don't Always Get It," *Prevention*, March 29, 2019, https://www.prevention.com/health/mental-health/a26678044/women-and-stress/.

Chapter 7: Energy Medicine 101

1 Romans 8:16, NIV.

2 Bruce Lipton, *The Biology of Belief*.

3 My good friend William Tiller, retired head of the physics department at Stanford, tells me that white paper #15 on his website gives credible scientific proof of how the Healing Codes and other energy modalities work, and that they do work. See William A Tiller, "White Papper XV. Preventative Medicine/Sefl-Healing via One's Personal Biofield Pumping and Blalancing," https://www.tillerinstitute.com/white_paper.html, accessed October 8, 2018. Also, the associated Cosortium of Energy Practitioners (ACEP), approved by the American Psychological Association to offer continuing education credits, has also compiled a list of abstracts of energy medicine studies. https://cdn.ymaws.com/www.energypsych.org/resource/resmgr/EP_Studies_with_Abstracts_by.pdf.

Chapter 8: Memory Engineering: You Have to See It to Believe It

1 Sandeep Joshi, "Memory Transference in Organ Transplant Patients," *Journal of New Approaches to Medicine and Health,* www.namahjournal.com/doc/Actual/Memory-transference-in-organ-transplant-recipients-vol-19-iss-1.html. Also see Marcus Lowth, "10 Organ Recipients Who Took on Traits of Their Donors," Listverse, listverse.com/2016/05/14/10-organ-recipients-who-took-on-the-traits-of-their-donors/; Lizette Borreli, "Can Organ Transplant Change a Recipient's Personality? Cell Memory Theory Affirms 'Yes,'" Medical Daily, www.medicaldaily.com/can-organ-transplant-change-recipients-personality-cell-memory-theory-affirms-yes-247498.

2 P. M. H. Atwater, "17 Near-Death Experiences That Changed Lives Positively," International Association for Near-Death Studies, Inc., iands.org/ndes/nde-stories/17-nde-accounts-from-beyond-the-light.html.

3 Ambrose, "A Cell Forgets."

4 Jason Castro, "The Era of Memory Engineering Has Arrived: How Neuroscientists Can Call Up and Change a Memory," *Scientific American,* July 30, 2013, www.scientificamerican.com/article/era-memory-engineering-has-arrived/.

5 Thanks to Lee Euler, publisher of the program Awakening from Alzheimer's, for sharing these virtual reality studies. Inbal Maidan, Keren Rosenberg-Katz, Yael Jacob, Nir Giladi, Jeffrey M. Hausdorff, and Anat Mirelman, "Disparate Effects of Training on Brain Activation in Parkinson Disease," *Neurology* 89, no. 17 (October 2017), 1804–1810; doi:10.1212/WNL.0000000000004576. Abstract available at www.ncbi.nlm.nih.gov/pubmed/28954877.

6 Ananya Bhattacharya, "Paraplegics Are Learning to Walk Again with Virtual Reality," Quartz, August 15, 2016, qz.com/757516/paraplegics-are-learning-to-walk-again-with-virtual-reality/.

7 Bhattacharya, "Paraplegics Are Learning to Walk Again with Virtual Reality." See also the original study: Ana R. C. Donati, Solaiman Shokur, Edgard Morya, Debora S. F. Campos, Renan C. Moioli, Claudia M. Gitti, Patricia B. Augusto, Sandra Tripodi, Cristhiane G. Pires, Gislaine A. Pereira, Fabricio L. Brasil, Simone Gallo, Anthony A. Lin, Angelo K. Takigami, Maria A. Aratanha, Sanjay Joshi, Hannes Bleuler, Gordon Cheng, Alan Rudolph, and Miguel A. L. Nicolelis, "Long-Term Training with a Brain-Machine Interface-Based Gait Protocol Induces Partial Neurological Recovery in Paraplegic Patients," *Scientific Reports,* August 11, 2016, www.nature.com/articles/srep30383, doi: doi.org/10.1038/srep30383.

8 Polona Pozeg, Estelle Palluel, Roberta Ronchi, Marco Solcà, Abdul-Wahab Al-Khodairy, Xavier Jordan, Ammar Kassouha, and Olaf Blanke, "Virtual Reality Improves Embodiment and Neuropathic Pain Caused by Spinal Cord Injury," *Neurology* 89, no. 18 (October 2017), 1894–1903; DOI:10.1212/WNL.0000000000004585. Abstract available at www.ncbi.nlm.nih.gov/pubmed/28986411.

9 I. Brunner, J. S. Skouen, H. Hofstad, J. Aßmus, F. Becker, A.M. Sanders, H. Pallesen, L. Qvist Kristensen, M. Michielsen, L. Thijs, and G. Verheyden, "Vir-

tual Reality Training for Upper Extremity in Subacute Stroke (VIRTUES): A Multicenter RCT," *Neurology* 89, no. 24 (2017), 2413–2421; doi: 10.1212/WNL.0000000000004744. Abstract available at www.ncbi.nlm.nih.gov/pubmed/29142090.

10 Caroline J. Falconer, Aitor Rovira, John A. King, Paul Gilbert, Angus Antley, Pasco Fearon, Neil Ralph, Mel Slater, and Chris R. Brewin, "Embodying Self-Compassion within Virtual Reality and Its Effects on Patients with Depression," *BJPsych Open* 2, no. 1 (2016): 74–80; doi:10.1192/bjpo.bp.115.002147. Abstract available at www.ncbi.nlm.nih.gov/pubmed/27703757.

11 Vartan C. Tashjian, Sasan Mosadeghi, Amber R. Howard, Mayra Lopez, Taylor Dupuy, Mark Reid, Bibiana Martinez, Shahzad Ahmed, Francis Dailey, Karen Robbins, Bradley Rosen, Garth Fuller, Itai Danovitch, Waguih IsHak, and Brennan Spiegel, "Virtual Reality for Management of Pain in Hospitalized Patients: Results of a Controlled Trial," *JMIR Mental Health* 4, no. 1 (2017), e9; doi: 10.2196/mental.7387. Abstract available at mental.jmir.org/2017/1/e9/.

12 Leonard Mlodinow, *Subliminal: How Your Unconscious Mind Rules Your Behavior*, 45.

ABOUT THE AUTHOR

Dr. Alexander Loyd, PhD, ND, is the international best-selling author of *The Love Code* and *The Healing Code*. He has been featured live on NBC, ABC, CBS, Fox, and PBS news programs as an expert in healing the source issues underlying disease and illness. Dr. Loyd lectures all over the world and has built the largest whole-life healing practice in the world, with hundreds of clients in fifty states and 172 countries (and counting). He lives in Tennessee with his wife, Hope, and sons, Harry and George.